The Simple Paleo

KITCHEN

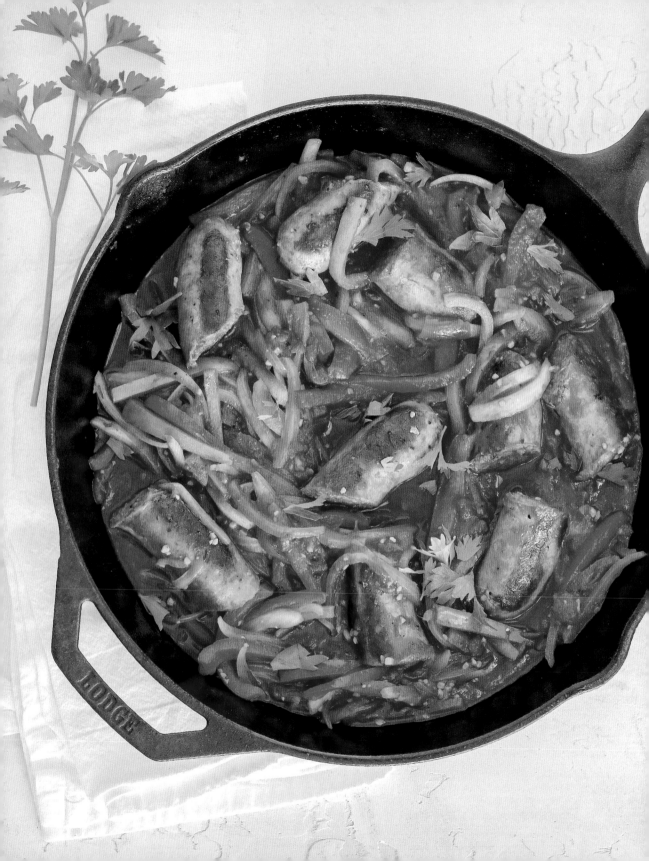

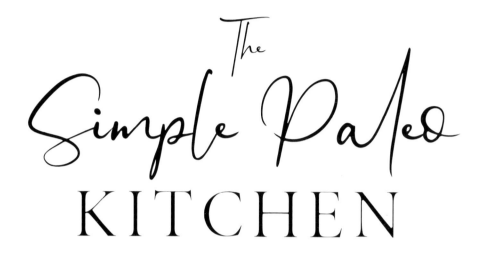

The Simple Paleo KITCHEN

60 DELICIOUS
GLUTEN- AND GRAIN-FREE
RECIPES WITHOUT
THE FUSS

Jessie Bittner

CREATOR OF JUST JESSIE B

PAGE STREET
PUBLISHING CO.

PAGE STREET
PUBLISHING CO.

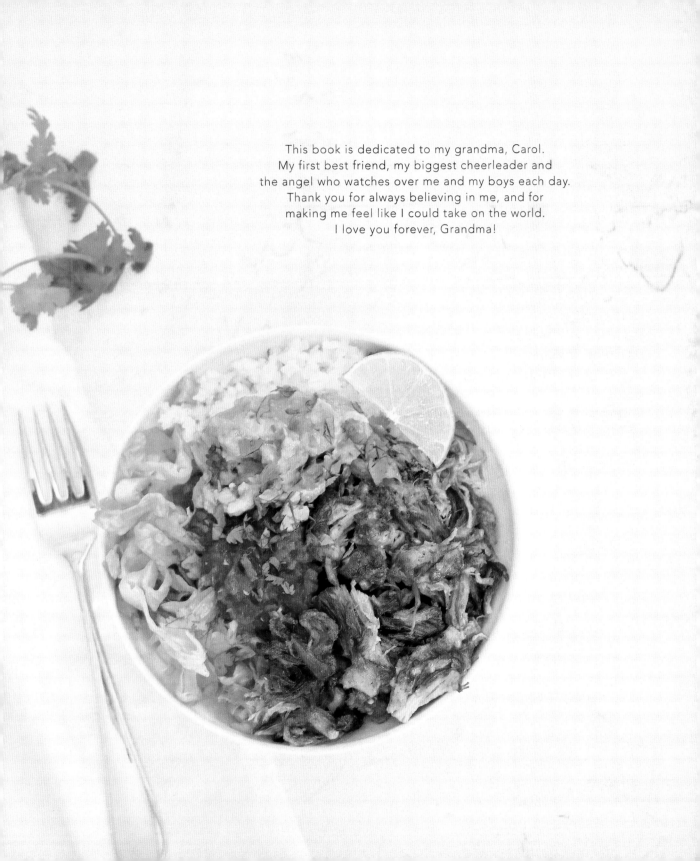

This book is dedicated to my grandma, Carol.
My first best friend, my biggest cheerleader and
the angel who watches over me and my boys each day.
Thank you for always believing in me, and for
making me feel like I could take on the world.
I love you forever, Grandma!

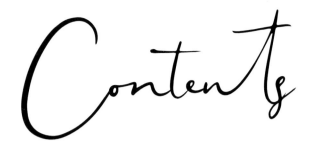

Contents

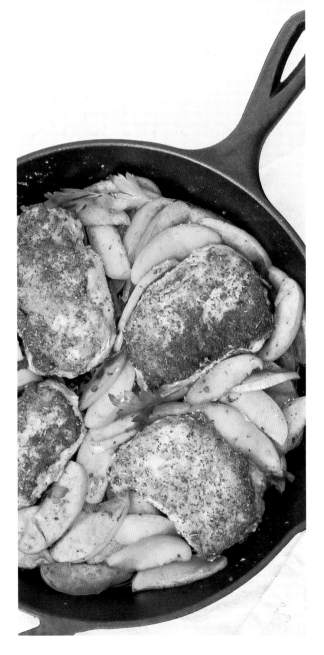

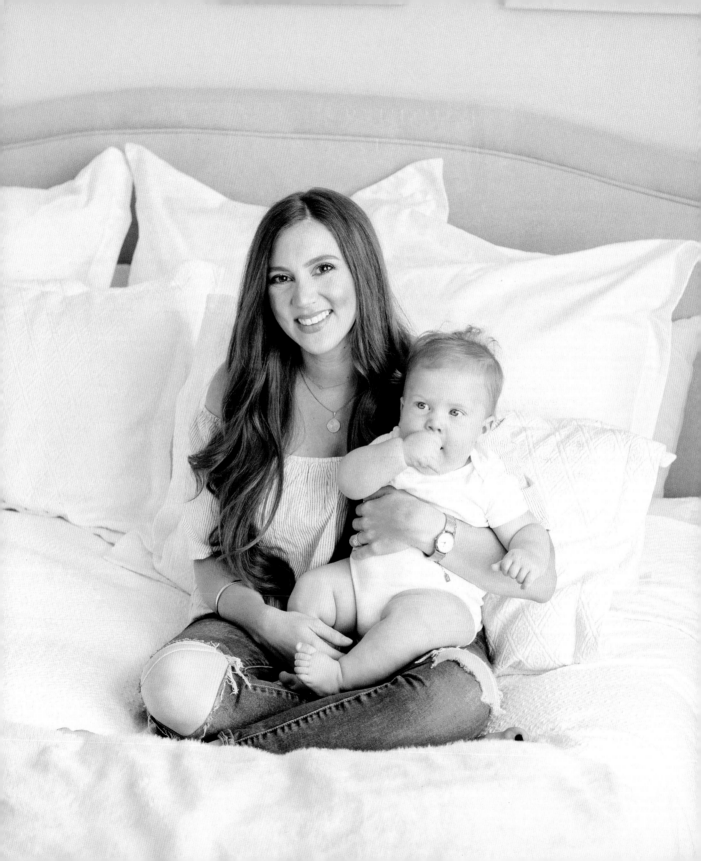

INTRODUCTION

By now, most of us know that real, simple, whole foods are generally the best for our health. Sounds easy, right? Yet once you get into the daily grind of cooking, cleaning, doing dishes and shopping—all while keeping the house together, bills paid and yourself and your family alive and well—the time and effort adds up, and it can feel overwhelming.

With this book, I want to share some of my favorite satisfying, family-friendly Paleo recipes that will leave you feeling your best—but without a sense of dread when it's time to be in the kitchen. Over my years of prioritizing healthy eating, tricks like prepping ahead, simplifying ingredient lists and minimizing dishes have kept me on track. My family is fed and happy, and I feel so good knowing that I'm fueling them with delicious whole foods that will love them back!

I found the Paleo diet eight years ago and was instantly hooked on how it made me feel. With the simple act of eliminating dairy, grains and refined sugars, the migraine headaches and "random" stomachaches I had suffered from for years went away. My skin glowed, my hair grew and maintaining a healthy weight felt effortless.

For years, I had felt like I was a "healthy eater." But let's just say that my so-called healthy diet wasn't always filled with real, whole foods. Low-fat, low-calorie and low-nutrient packaged foods were convenient, and marketing made me feel like I was making good choices, but the way I felt physically wasn't reflecting a healthy lifestyle.

I met my husband in grad school, and he introduced me to a new way of looking at food. The Paleo diet reframed my thinking as I started prioritizing nutrition over convenience: I began looking at food as fuel and finding ways to make simple, whole foods taste delicious and fit my budget and time constraints.

As a busy grad student working toward my master's degree, I spent all day working at internships and all night taking classes, commuting home and studying until I couldn't keep my eyes open. I was exhausted, but I knew that good food would help me be my best—so I made it my priority. I cooked in batches each week, carried a cooler bag brimming with breakfast, lunch, snacks and dinner with me each day and ate my salads and homemade chili in the back row of my night classes.

Nowadays, I'm a busy, self-employed, work-from-home wife and mom of a rambunctious toddler and a baby. I have found myself whittling down the "fuss" and "fluff" in the kitchen even further — to just what's really necessary. I make breakfasts ahead so my family and I can grab and go, have small bites on hand for quick lunches and snacks and put the Instant Pot® and slow cooker to work on simple recipes that make plenty of servings. I keep the same pantry staples on hand each week and am constantly reinventing them into new dishes that don't require daily grocery trips. One-dish meals are my thing, and any dish or pan that can get covered in parchment paper to reduce kitchen cleanup does.

Regardless of how quick and easy my recipes have become, one thing has remained: flavor that is far from simple! I am a foodie at heart, my husband loves to eat and I want to feed my boys the delicious comfort foods that I grew up on. But above all, I want my family to feel our best every day and truly thrive—and that is what eating a Paleo diet has done for us.

This book takes you down the path that's led to the most sustainability for me when it comes to true health: simple, delicious Paleo recipes that make the most of your time in the kitchen.

I truly hope you enjoy these recipes, from my kitchen and family to yours.

XO,

Jessie

Jessie Bittner

PALEO PANTRY STAPLES

When it comes to my fridge and pantry, I like to keep things simple! The following list doesn't include everything, but it does cover most of the key players in the Paleo recipes that I make on a day-to-day basis.

PANTRY STAPLES

Almond and coconut milk: I use unsweetened, unflavored dairy-free milks in many of my recipes to help add creaminess or to thin sauces or batters. Most recipes can be made with boxed or refrigerated cartons of milk—the varieties that are on the thinner side. Be sure to double-check the ingredients for weird additives (e.g., soy lecithin, sulfites, carrageenan) or hidden sugars. For some recipes, I call for full-fat coconut milk, which can be purchased in a shelf-stable can.

Chocolate chips: Look for dairy-free chocolate chips. My favorite brand for chips and chunks of all kinds is Enjoy Life. Chopping up a chocolate bar made with simple ingredients is another great option.

Coconut aminos: This is the soy-free and gluten-free alternative to soy sauce that I love for its salty, smoky, savory flavor. You can find it at most grocery stores now, near the soy sauce or Asian foods.

Cooking spray: Avocado or olive oil spray comes in handy for greasing a dish or for lightly coating vegetables with fat. I look for sprays that list oil as the only ingredient. You can always substitute a light drizzle of avocado or olive oil if you don't have cooking spray.

Grain-free flours: You can always find my pantry stocked with almond, arrowroot, coconut and tapioca flours. Grain-free flours are tricky and often not interchangeable (at least not on a 1:1 ratio). Keep these flours on hand, and try buying them in bulk online like I do!

Ghee: I use this interchangeably with butter in just about any recipe. If you can tolerate grass-fed butter, I love the texture. But if you're sensitive to dairy, ghee might be a great option for you since it is clarified, meaning the milk solids are removed. If ghee is also a no-go for you, see the particular recipe you want to make for other options (coconut and avocado oil can often be substituted, depending on the recipe).

Mayo: I am not a "mayo person," but I love employing it to add creaminess to certain sauces and dishes. I look for mayo that has clean, simple ingredients, no added sugar and uses a good-quality oil like avocado oil.

Nut butters: I often use creamy nut butters for everything from baking to dressings. Almond butter and cashew butter are my favorites, but sunflower butter can be substituted if you have a nut allergy. Coconut butter has a great texture and can be found online or in health food stores. I buy organic nut butters when I can, and I look for the fewest possible ingredients.

Nutritional yeast: This inactive yeast adds a savory, nutty, cheesy flavor and thickens liquids as well. This is one of my "secret ingredients" that brings many soups and sauces together and adds an element of flavor that I love but that isn't easily identifiable. Look for nutritional yeast in the bulk section at your grocery store, or grab some online.

Raw cashews: I use these in baking, but I also love them for thickening sauces and soups. They have a mild, creamy flavor and make a great swap for heavy cream when blended with liquid. I purchase them in bulk and always have some on hand.

Shredded coconut: Look for unsweetened shredded coconut, sometimes called desiccated coconut. It's the finely shredded stuff about the size of grains of rice or smaller. Shredded coconut adds great texture and flavor to sweet and savory dishes alike.

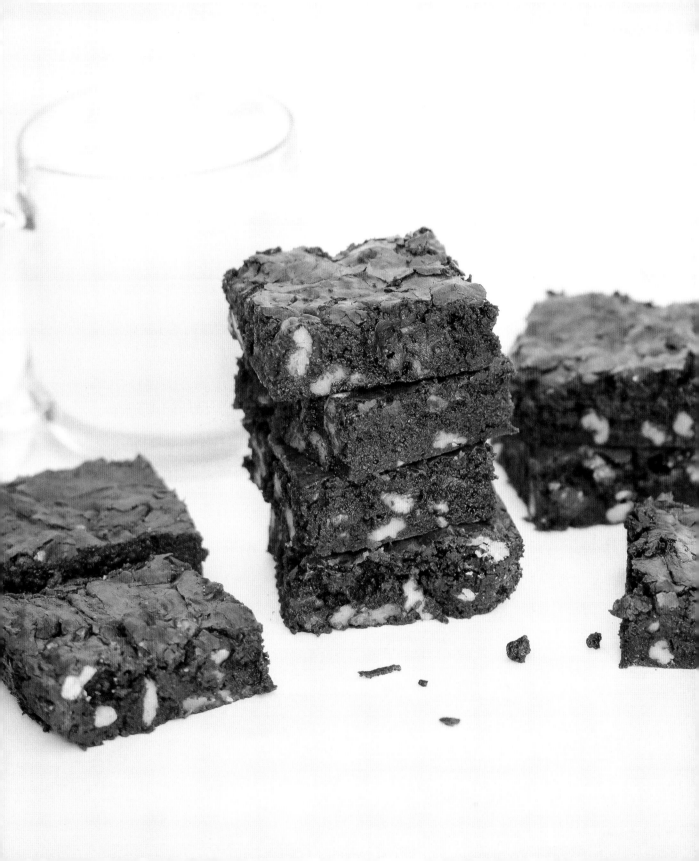

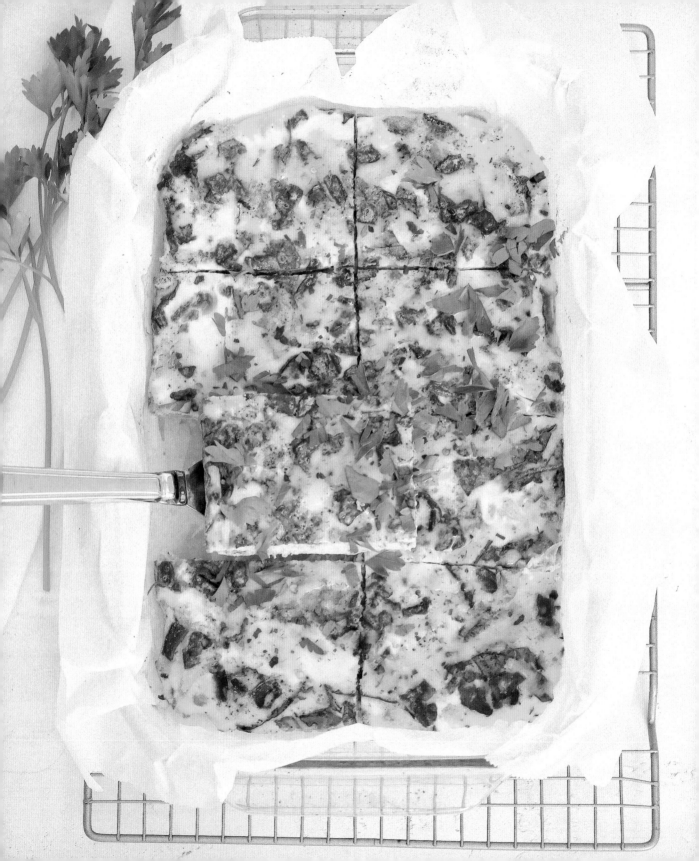

Make-Ahead Breakfasts

Breakfast is often called the most important meal of the day, but it can also be the trickiest if you're not prepared. Whether it's savory or sweet, make it the easiest meal of the day by taking some time to batch-cook ahead of time. I like to make breakfasts on Sundays, enjoy a portion that day and save the rest for throughout the week. The freezer is another great option if you won't eat the whole dish quickly enough—just reheat and serve leftovers whenever you're ready! My general rule is to store food in the fridge for 4 to 5 days or in the freezer for about 3 months.

BREAKFAST BURRITO BOWLS WITH SPICY RANCH

There's nothing more satisfying than a savory breakfast burrito stuffed with crispy potatoes, tender peppers and onions and some fluffy scrambled eggs laced with sausage. We're serving it up bowl-style here to keep it simple for an easy meal prep that's also great for entertaining!

YIELD: 4 SERVINGS

1 lb (454 g) ground pork breakfast sausage

4 tbsp (60 ml) avocado oil or melted ghee, divided

¼ cup (60 ml) unsweetened coconut milk

12 large eggs, beaten

½ tsp salt

¼ tsp black pepper

¼ cup (25 g) thinly sliced green onions

½ medium red bell pepper, diced

½ medium sweet onion, diced

2 medium Russet potatoes, cooked and cut into bite-size pieces

Chopped fresh cilantro, as needed (optional)

Fresh salsa, as needed (optional)

SPICY RANCH

½ cup (120 ml) Quick Homemade Ranch (page 123) or store-bought Paleo ranch dressing

2 tsp (10 ml) hot sauce, plus more as needed

1. In a large skillet over medium-high heat, cook the sausage for about 7 minutes, until the meat is browned and crumbled into small pieces. Drain the fat from the skillet, transfer the sausage to a medium bowl and set the bowl aside.

2. Reduce the heat to medium. Add 2 tablespoons (30 ml) of the oil to the skillet and heat the oil until it is warm. Whisk the coconut milk into the eggs and season the mixture with the salt and black pepper. Pour the eggs into the skillet and cook them for 4 to 5 minutes, until they are fluffy and scrambled, stirring occasionally to ensure they cook evenly. Stir the sausage and green onions into the eggs and set the skillet aside.

3. In a separate large skillet over medium heat, heat 1 tablespoon (15 ml) of the oil. Add the bell pepper and onion, and sauté the vegetables for 4 to 5 minutes, or until they are tender. Scoot the vegetables to the side of the skillet, increase the heat to medium-high and add the remaining 1 tablespoon (15 ml) of oil to the center of the skillet. Add the potatoes and cook them for 7 to 10 minutes, or until the potatoes are golden brown. Stir the potatoes and vegetables together.

4. To make the Spicy Ranch, in a small bowl, combine the Quick Homemade Ranch and hot sauce, stirring the mixture until it is smooth.

5. Assemble the burrito bowls with a scoop of the egg and sausage mixture and a scoop of the potato mixture. Top each bowl with a drizzle of the Spicy Ranch, the cilantro (if using) and the salsa (if using). Store prepped meals in airtight containers in the refrigerator for 4 to 5 days.

NOTE: Keep baked Russet or sweet potatoes on hand for meals like this. They reduce the cooking time, and they get extra crispy because they've been cooked twice!

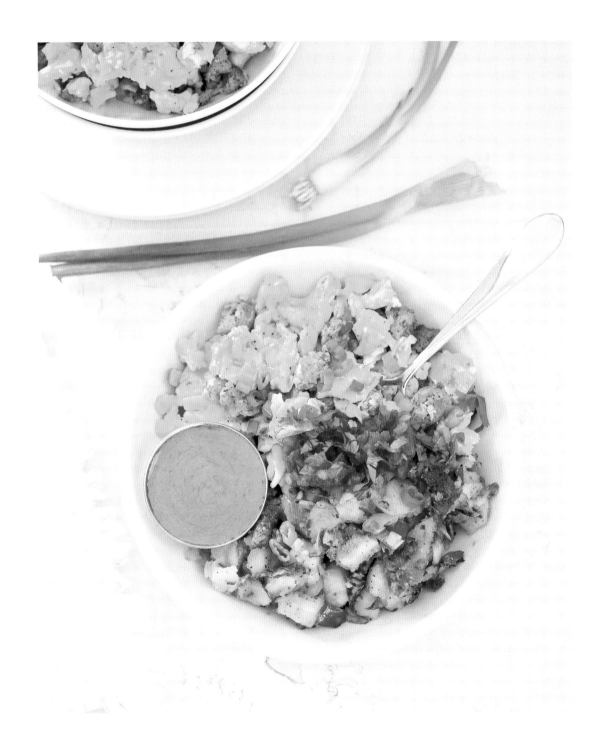

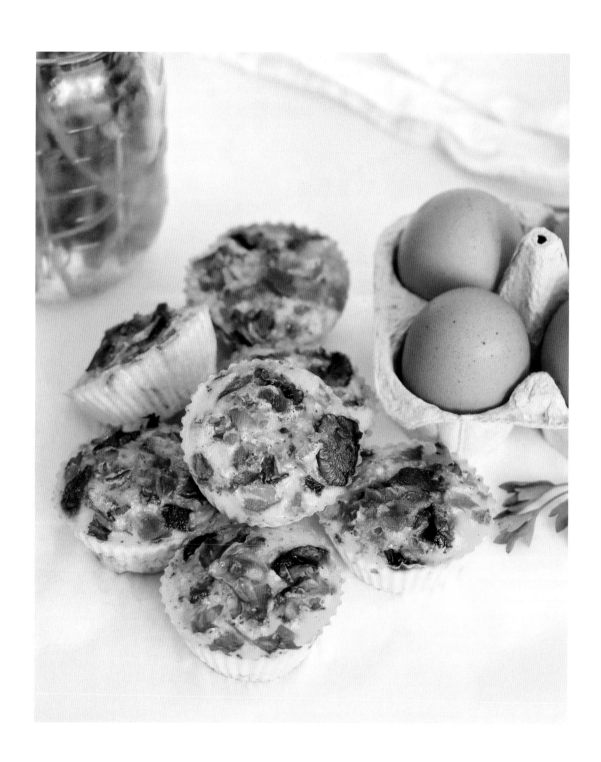

BACON AND VEGGIE EGG BITES

Nothing says "grab-and-go breakfast" like these protein- and flavor-packed egg bites. Fill them with your favorite veggies and crispy bacon, and bake them until they're set. Store them in the fridge and simply reheat one for an easy morning bite that will keep you full and satisfied!

YIELD: 12 BITES

12 large eggs

½ tsp garlic powder

¼ tsp salt

¼ tsp black pepper

6 slices cooked bacon, roughly chopped

¼ cup (17 g) finely chopped cremini mushrooms

¼ cup (44 g) diced red bell pepper

1 tbsp (4 g) finely chopped fresh parsley

1. Preheat the oven to 350°F (177°C). Line a 12-well muffin pan with parchment paper liners.

2. In a large bowl, whisk together the eggs, garlic powder, salt and black pepper. Fill each muffin well halfway with the egg mixture. Divide the bacon, mushrooms, bell pepper and parsley evenly among the wells.

3. Bake the egg bites for 20 minutes, or until the eggs are set.

4. Serve the egg bites hot, or store them in an airtight container in the refrigerator for 4 to 5 days and reheat them when you are ready to serve.

NOTE: To freeze, wrap each egg bite in plastic wrap or parchment paper and then wrap again with a layer of aluminum foil. To reheat, allow the egg bites to fully thaw in the refrigerator overnight. Bake them at 350°F (177°C) for about 10 minutes, or until warmed through.

OVERNIGHT SLOW COOKER BREAKFAST CASSEROLE

This hearty breakfast is my favorite for entertaining. Set it the night before, and let the magic happen overnight. Wake up to the smells of savory sausage, bacon and potatoes ready for everyone—or even just you—to enjoy. The crisp crust and fluffy center of this casserole cannot be beat!

YIELD: 8 SERVINGS

1 lb (454 g) ground pork breakfast sausage

Avocado oil or melted ghee, as needed

1 lb (454 g) fresh or frozen shredded potatoes

1 medium red bell pepper, diced

⅓ cup (33 g) thinly sliced green onions

6 to 8 slices of bacon, roughly chopped

16 large eggs

½ cup (120 ml) unsweetened coconut or almond milk

1 tsp garlic powder

½ tsp salt

½ tsp black pepper

1. In a large skillet over medium-high heat, cook the sausage for about 7 minutes, until the sausage is crumbly and browned. Drain the fat from the skillet and set the sausage aside.

2. Grease the bottom and sides of the slow cooker insert well with the oil. Add the potatoes to the insert, pressing them down slightly to pack them in. Top the potatoes with the sausage, bell pepper, green onions and bacon.

3. In a large bowl, whisk together the eggs, milk, garlic powder, salt and black pepper. Pour the egg mixture over the meat and vegetable mixture.

4. Cook the casserole on low for 6 to 8 hours. Set the slow cooker to warm once the casserole has finished cooking, and serve when you're ready.

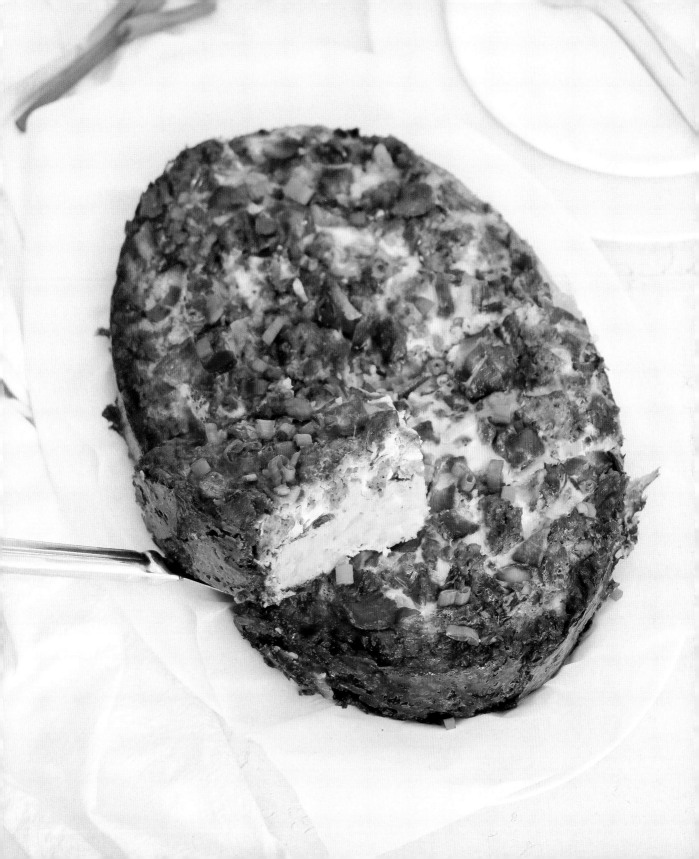

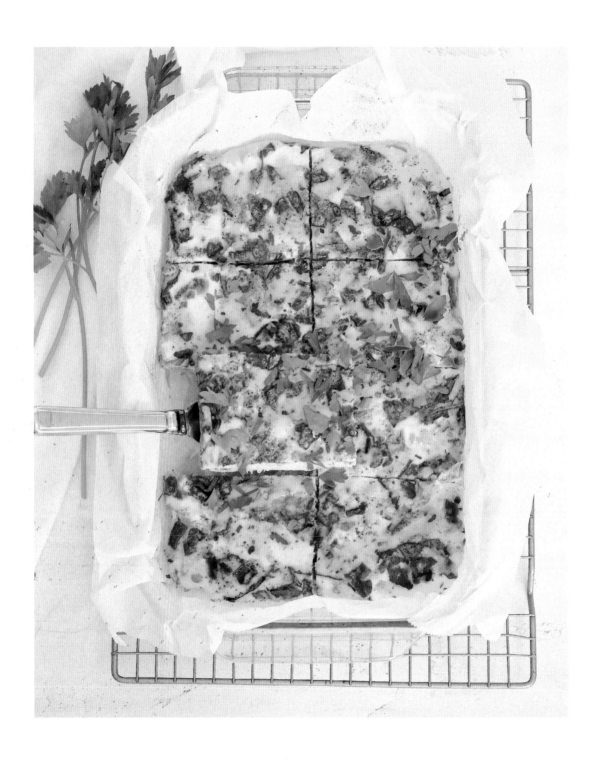

CHICKEN-BACON-RANCH BREAKFAST BAKE

A classic comfort food combo: chicken, bacon, ranch! Here it's done breakfast style in a savory bake you can make on a Sunday and enjoy all week long. Rotisserie chicken or leftovers from cooked chicken breasts or thighs work great for this recipe to cut down on time.

YIELD: 6 TO 8 SERVINGS

12 large eggs

¼ cup (60 ml) unsweetened coconut or almond milk

1 tsp onion powder

1 tsp garlic powder

½ tsp salt

½ tsp black pepper

½ tsp dried dill

8 slices of bacon, divided

2 to 3 cups (250 to 375 g) shredded cooked chicken

1 cup (30 g) baby spinach, roughly chopped

Roughly chopped fresh parsley, as needed (optional)

Quick Homemade Ranch (page 123), as needed (optional)

1. Preheat the oven to 375°F (191°C). Line a 9 x 13–inch (23 x 33–cm) glass baking dish with parchment paper. Set it aside.

2. In a large bowl, whisk together the eggs, milk, onion powder, garlic powder, salt, black pepper and dill.

3. Chop 6 slices of the bacon and set them aside for the breakfast bake filling. Chop the remaining 2 slices of bacon and set them aside for topping the breakfast bake. Place the chicken, 6 slices of chopped bacon and spinach in the prepared baking dish. Pour the egg mixture over the chicken mixture, and top the breakfast bake with the remaining bacon.

4. Bake the casserole for 35 minutes, or until the eggs are set. Garnish the breakfast bake with the parsley (if using) and Quick Homemade Ranch (if using), and serve the breakfast bake warm.

NOTE: Leftovers can be stored in the refrigerator in an airtight container for 4 to 5 days and reheated when you're ready to serve. To freeze, wrap individual servings in plastic wrap or parchment paper, then wrap again with aluminum foil before placing in the freezer. To reheat, allow the slices to fully thaw in the refrigerator overnight. Bake at 350°F (177°C) for about 10 minutes, or until warmed through.

CHORIZO AND SWEET POTATO SHEET PAN BREAKFAST

Perfect for making ahead, this sheet pan breakfast is packed with mouthwatering spicy flavors from the chorizo yet is balanced with the sweetness of roasted red bell peppers and tender sweet potatoes. My family loves to load this one with lots of garnishes, and sometimes we even serve it with a fried or poached egg on top!

YIELD: 8 SERVINGS

3 small sweet potatoes, cut into ½" (13-mm) pieces

2 medium red bell peppers, cut into ½" (13-mm) pieces

2 tbsp (30 ml) avocado oil

½ tsp garlic powder

½ tsp salt

¼ tsp black pepper

1 lb (454 g) ground chorizo sausage, cut into bite-size pieces

Thinly sliced avocado, as needed (optional)

Finely chopped fresh cilantro, as needed (optional)

Thinly sliced jalapeño, as needed (optional)

Lime wedges, as needed (optional)

1. Preheat the oven to 350°F (177°C). In a large bowl, toss the sweet potatoes and bell peppers with the oil, garlic powder, salt and black pepper. Spread the mixture out on a large, rimmed baking sheet.

2. Add the chorizo pieces to the mixture, tucking them in evenly among the vegetables.

3. Bake the mixture for 45 minutes, or until the sausage is cooked through and the sweet potatoes are tender and lightly browned.

4. Garnish the sheet pan breakfast with the avocado (if using), cilantro (if using), jalapeño (if using) and a squeeze of fresh lime juice from the lime wedges (if using), then serve.

NOTE: Leftovers can be stored in the refrigerator in an airtight container for 4 to 5 days and reheated when you're ready to serve.

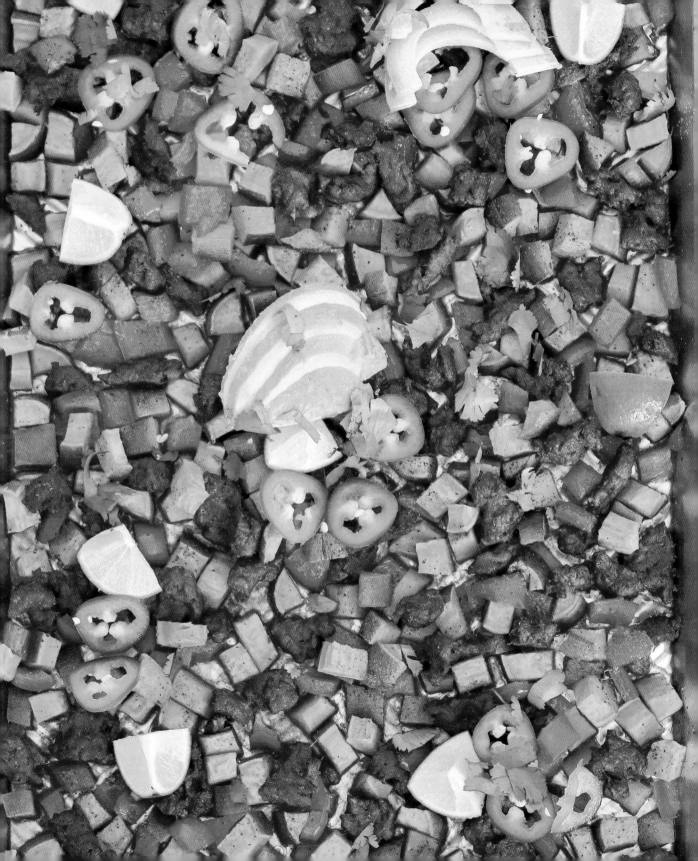

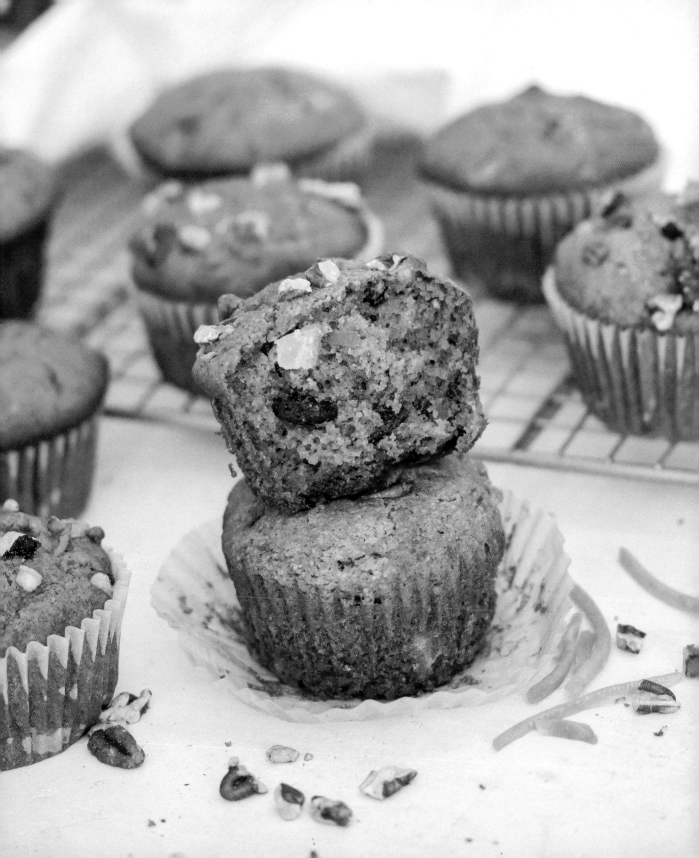

MORNING GLORY MUFFINS

If apple-cinnamon spice cake and carrot cake had a baby, it would be these warm and hearty muffins. They are full of warm spices and healthy fats, and they're extra filling with diced apples, shredded carrots, raisins and pecans. Try these as a quick, nutritious on-the-go breakfast, or freeze a batch to keep on hand for breakfast emergencies!

YIELD: 12 MUFFINS

3 large eggs

⅓ cup (60 g) cashew or almond butter

½ cup (25 g) shredded carrots

½ cup (60 g) diced apples (any variety)

⅓ cup (80 ml) honey

3 tbsp (45 g) coconut oil or ghee, melted

1 tsp pure vanilla extract

2 cups (192 g) almond flour

½ cup (61 g) pecans, roughly chopped

⅓ cup (50 g) raisins

2 tsp (6 g) ground cinnamon

½ tsp ground nutmeg

1 tsp baking soda

½ tsp salt

1. Preheat the oven to 350°F (177°C). Line a 12-well muffin pan with parchment paper liners.

2. In a large bowl, combine the eggs, cashew butter, carrots, apples, honey, oil and vanilla, stirring until the mixture is smooth.

3. Add the flour, pecans, raisins, cinnamon, nutmeg, baking soda and salt and stir until the ingredients are just combined.

4. Scoop the batter into the prepared muffin pan, filling each well up about three-fourths of the way. Bake the muffins for 20 to 25 minutes, or until a toothpick inserted into the center of a muffin comes out clean.

5. Let the muffins cool in the muffin pan for 5 minutes before transferring the muffins to a cooling rack. Allow the muffins to cool fully, then store them at room temperature, covered loosely with a cloth or paper towel.

NOTE: To freeze these muffins, wrap each cooled muffin with plastic wrap or parchment paper and then again with aluminum foil. To reheat, allow the muffins to fully thaw in the refrigerator overnight. Bake at 350°F (177°C) for 8 to 10 minutes, or until they are warmed through.

SWEET CINNAMON GRANOLA

This grain-free spin on sweet, crunchy granola fills every cereal need I've ever had. Enjoy it by the handful when you need a little somethin' on top of a smoothie bowl, or serve it like a traditional cereal with chilled coconut or almond milk. Make this big batch and keep it on hand for easy meals and snacks anytime!

YIELD: 8 CUPS (1.9 KG)

½ cup (90 g) cashew or almond butter

½ cup (120 ml) pure maple syrup

⅓ cup (80 g) coconut oil, melted

2 tsp (10 ml) pure vanilla extract

1 tbsp (9 g) ground cinnamon

1 cup (110 g) sliced almonds

½ cup (63 g) roughly chopped pecans

½ cup (75 g) roughly chopped raw cashews

½ cup (38 g) unsweetened shredded coconut

½ cup (48 g) almond flour

½ tsp salt

1. Preheat the oven to 350°F (177°C). Line a large baking sheet with parchment paper.

2. In a large bowl, combine the cashew butter, maple syrup, oil, vanilla and cinnamon, stirring until the mixture is smooth. Add the almonds, pecans, cashews, coconut, flour and salt, and stir until the ingredients are combined. Spread the mixture evenly onto the prepared baking sheet.

3. Bake the granola for 15 minutes, or until it is golden brown but not burned on the edges. Allow the granola to cool completely before using your hands to break it into crumbles.

4. Store the granola in an airtight container in a cool, dark place for up to 4 weeks.

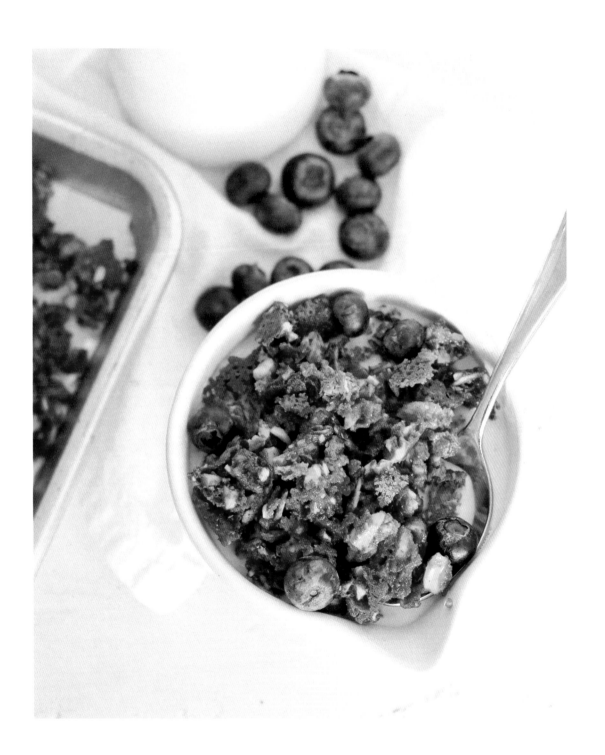

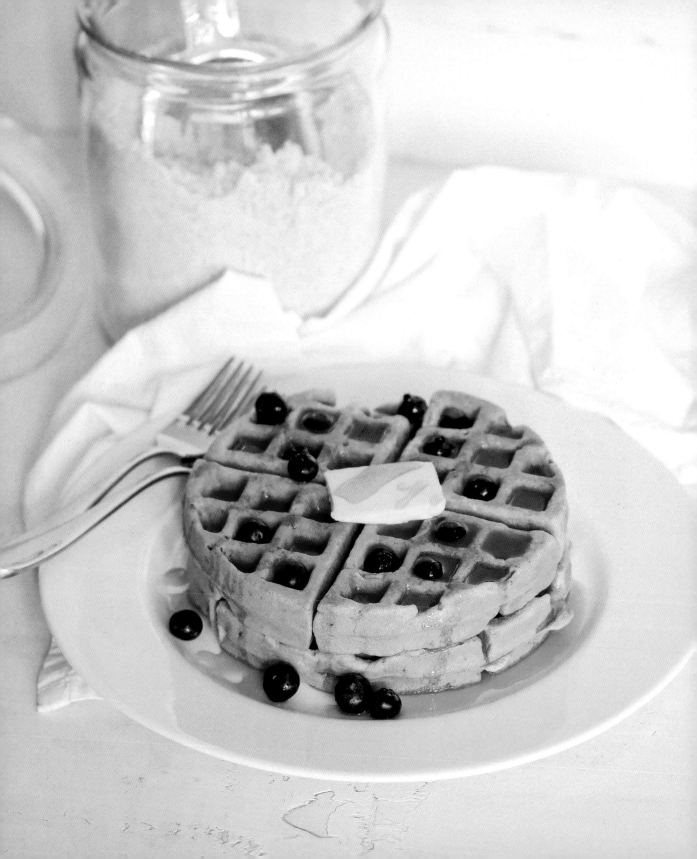

FLUFFY PANCAKE AND WAFFLE MIX

Sunday mornings in our home are always slow and include pancakes or waffles for the whole family. This mix is our go-to for speeding up the process, and it makes the fluffiest pancakes and waffles that are sweet and filling. While this recipe makes just one batch of mix, I recommend making a triple batch—or more—of the dry mix ahead of time. Or try freezing your finished pancakes and waffles for a quick breakfast you can reheat in the morning.

YIELD: 10 (4-INCH [10-CM]) PANCAKES, OR 4 LARGE WAFFLES

(yield may vary depending on the size of the waffle iron used)

DRY PANCAKE AND WAFFLE MIX

½ cup (48 g) almond flour

⅓ cup (42 g) tapioca flour

¼ cup (32 g) coconut flour

¼ cup (48 g) coconut sugar

½ tsp baking soda

¼ tsp salt

PANCAKES OR WAFFLES

4 large eggs

¼ cup (60 ml) unsweetened almond or coconut milk

1 tsp apple cider vinegar

1 tsp pure vanilla extract

Ghee or coconut oil, as needed (for pancakes only)

Pure maple syrup, as needed

Fresh fruit, as needed

1. To prepare the dry pancake or waffle mix, combine the almond flour, tapioca flour, coconut flour, sugar, baking soda and salt in a medium bowl.

2. When you are ready to use the dry mix, whisk the eggs in a medium bowl. Stir in the almond milk, vinegar and vanilla. Add the egg mixture to the flour mixture and whisk until the batter is smooth.

3. To make pancakes, heat a large skillet or griddle over medium heat and coat it with the ghee. Pour about ¼ cup (60 ml) of batter into the skillet. Cook the pancake for 2 to 3 minutes, then flip it and cook it for 1 to 2 minutes, or until it is light golden brown on each side.

4. To make waffles, heat a waffle iron to medium heat. Fill the iron with batter, and cook the waffle per the waffle iron's instructions until it is golden on the outside and cooked through in the center.

5. Serve the pancakes or waffles warm with the maple syrup and fruit. Keep extra pancakes or waffles in the refrigerator for up to 1 week, or store them wrapped in plastic in the freezer for up to 3 months.

NOTE: Try making the dry mix in bulk and saving it in an airtight container in the pantry. When you're ready to make pancakes or waffles, measure out 1½ cups (360 g) of dry mix for one batch of the recipe.

BANANA-BLUEBERRY BREAKFAST BREAD

A simple banana bread gets a flavor boost from fresh blueberries and makes the perfect morning bite. Keep slices in the fridge for a midmorning snack or as part of an easy breakfast with some protein like hard-boiled eggs or my Bacon and Veggie Egg Bites (page 19). If you're craving something extra sweet, try substituting Paleo-friendly chocolate chips for the blueberries!

YIELD: 6 TO 8 SLICES

2 medium overripe bananas, mashed

2 large eggs, at room temperature

3 tbsp (45 g) coconut oil, melted and cooled

3 tbsp (45 ml) honey or pure maple syrup

1 tsp pure vanilla extract

2 cups (192 g) almond flour

1 tsp baking powder

½ tsp salt

1 cup (150 g) fresh blueberries, divided

1. Preheat the oven to 350°F (177°C). Line a 9 x 5–inch (23 x 13–cm) loaf pan with parchment paper.

2. In a large bowl, combine the bananas, eggs, oil, honey and vanilla. Stir in the flour, baking powder and salt. Gently fold in ½ cup (75 g) of the blueberries.

3. Transfer the batter into the prepared loaf pan and sprinkle the remaining ½ cup (75 g) of blueberries on top. Bake the bread for 45 to 60 minutes, or until it is golden brown and firm in the center.

4. Allow the bread to cool, then slice it and serve. Store the remaining bread, covered with a paper towel, at room temperature for up to 2 days. If you do not eat the bread within that time, keep it in the refrigerator in an airtight container for 4 to 5 days.

NOTE: To make this recipe as muffins, scoop the batter into a lined 12-well muffin pan, then sprinkle the remaining ½ cup (75 g) of blueberries on top. Bake the muffins at 350°F (177°C) for 25 minutes, or until they are firm.

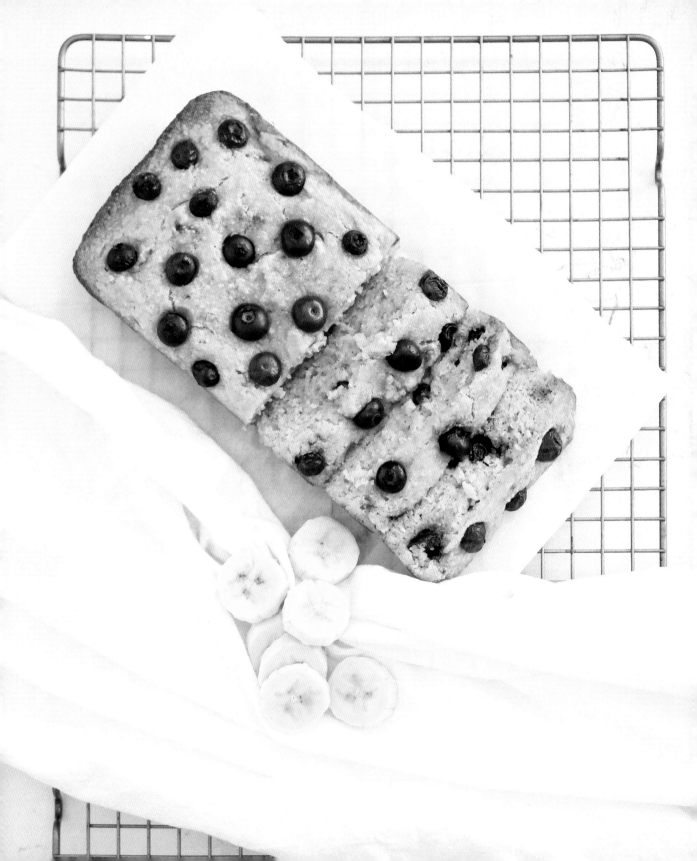

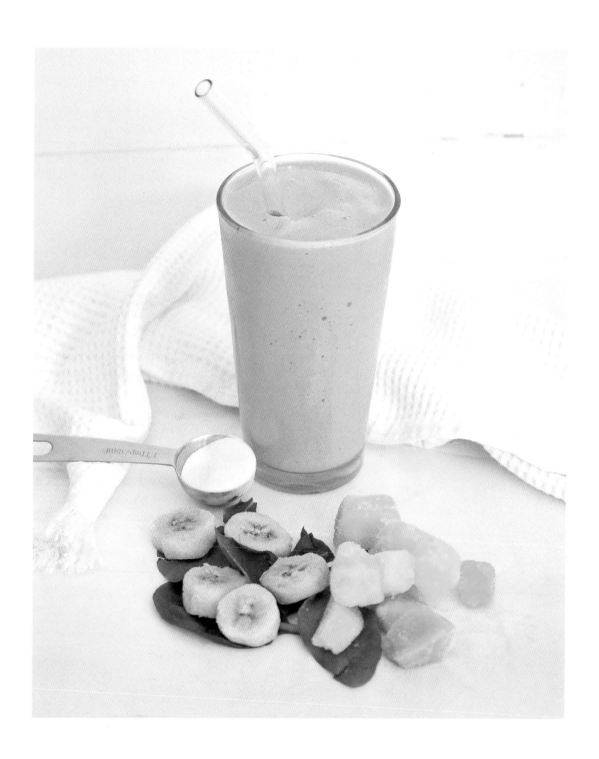

TROPICAL GREEN SMOOTHIE PACKS

Smoothies are an easy way to consume lots of nutrients really fast, and they're perfect for a busy morning's breakfast. These prep-ahead smoothie packs make it even quicker to get a great meal: Store them in the freezer and blend when you're ready. I add collagen peptides or a Paleo-friendly protein powder and 1 tablespoon (15 g) of coconut butter for healthy fats and an amped-up tropical flavor!

YIELD: 1 SERVING

SMOOTHIE PACK

½ cup (83 g) pineapple chunks

½ cup (83 g) mango chunks

½ cup (75 g) banana slices

2 cups (60 g) baby spinach or baby kale

SMOOTHIE

1 tbsp (15 g) coconut butter or coconut oil (optional)

1 scoop collagen peptides or protein powder of choice

1 to 1½ cups (240 to 360 ml) liquid of choice (see Note)

3 drops liquid stevia or 1 tsp pure maple syrup (optional)

½ tsp pure vanilla extract (optional)

1. To prepare the smoothie pack, combine the pineapple, mango, banana and spinach in a freezer-safe bag. Transfer the smoothie pack to the freezer and freeze until the contents are frozen solid. Store the smoothie pack in the freezer for up to 3 months.

2. To make the smoothie, empty the contents of the smoothie pack into a blender. Add the coconut butter, collagen peptides, liquid of choice, liquid stevia (if using) and vanilla (if using).

3. Blend the ingredients until they are smooth.

NOTE: My personal preference is to use 1¼ cups (300 ml) of liquid. I use ½ cup (120 ml) of coconut milk and ¾ cup (180 ml) of water or coconut water. If you prefer thicker smoothies, use 1 cup (240 ml) of liquid; if you prefer thinner smoothies, use 1½ cups (360 ml) of liquid.

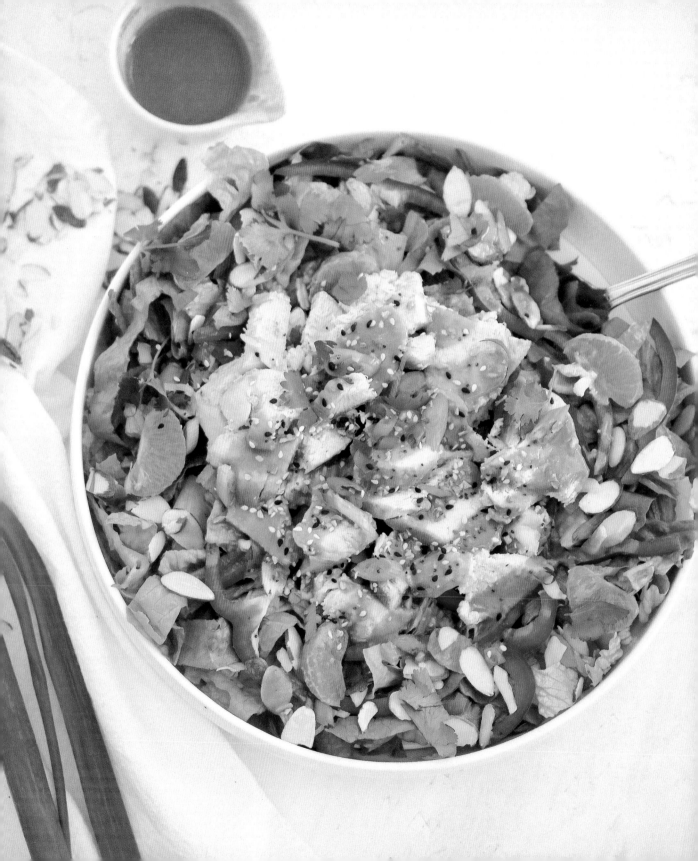

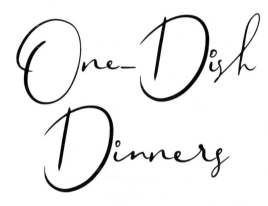

One-Dish Dinners

Kitchen cleanup is never fun, but it's especially annoying on a busy night when you want to eat a delicious meal and then be done. This chapter is all about the beauty of one-dish meals: Whether they're cooked in a skillet, pot, bowl or on a baking sheet, these recipes come together with just one main dish. Any prep items, such as cutting boards and small bowls, can be washed while the main meal cooks.

Keep it simple yet flavorful and fun, and minimize those dishes!

CREAMY LEMON-BUTTER CHICKEN SKILLET

Crispy pan-seared chicken is smothered in a mouthwatering, creamy lemon-butter sauce with some handfuls of fresh spinach for good measure. It's fresh and bright yet hearty and comforting all at once. Serve the chicken on its own or over smashed red or gold potatoes to bulk the dish up a bit.

YIELD: 6 SERVINGS

6 medium bone-in, skin-on chicken thighs

1 tbsp (9 g) smoked paprika

Salt, as needed

Black pepper, as needed

4 tbsp (60 g) grass-fed butter or ghee, divided

2 tsp (6 g) minced garlic

1 cup (240 ml) chicken broth

½ cup (120 ml) full-fat coconut milk

¼ cup (43 g) nutritional yeast

Zest of 1 medium lemon

Juice of 1 medium lemon

1 tsp Italian seasoning

2 cups (30 g) baby spinach, roughly chopped

1. Preheat the oven to 400°F (204°C). Season both sides of the chicken thighs with the paprika, salt and black pepper.

2. Melt 2 tablespoons (30 g) of the butter in a large ovenproof skillet over medium-high heat. Once the butter is hot, add the chicken, skin side down, and sear each side for 2 to 3 minutes, until each side is golden brown. Remove the chicken thighs from the skillet and set them aside. Drain the fat from the skillet, then return the skillet to the heat and melt the remaining 2 tablespoons (30 g) of butter.

3. Add the garlic and cook it for 1 to 2 minutes, or until it is just golden and fragrant. Stir in the broth, coconut milk, nutritional yeast, lemon zest, lemon juice and Italian seasoning.

4. Stir in the spinach, then bring the mixture to a simmer and cook it for 3 to 5 minutes, until the spinach has wilted and the sauce has slightly thickened. Add the chicken back to the skillet.

5. Transfer the skillet to the oven and bake the chicken for 25 to 30 minutes, or until the chicken's internal temperature is 165°F (74°C). Serve the chicken hot.

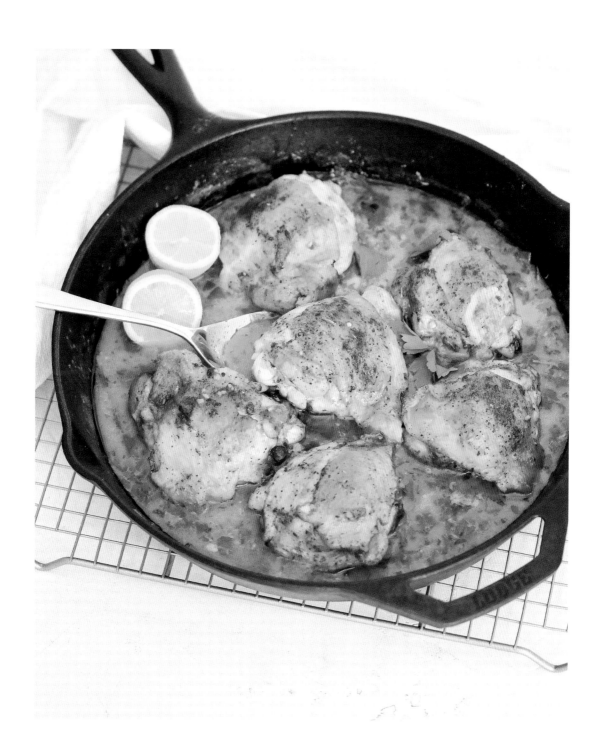

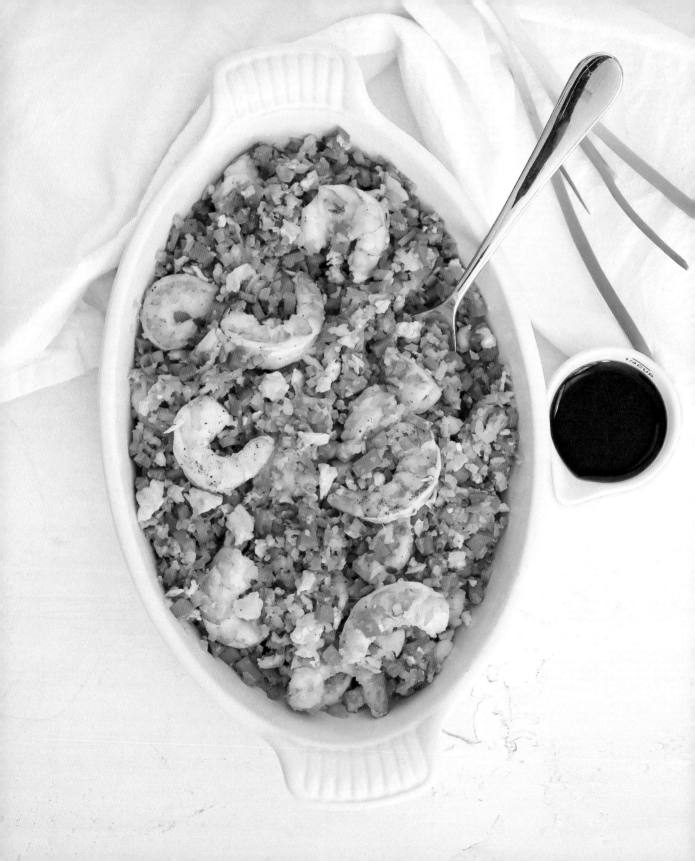

TAKEOUT-STYLE SHRIMP FRIED RICE

When fried rice is this easy and tastes this good, there's no reason for takeout. Make this one-dish meal in fewer than fifteen minutes, and enjoy it anytime you have a craving for Chinese takeout. It's veggie-packed and full of savory flavor you'll want to experience again and again!

YIELD: 4 SERVINGS

1 lb (454 g) large fresh or thawed frozen shrimp, peeled and deveined

Salt, as needed

Black pepper, as needed

2 tbsp (30 ml) avocado or coconut oil, divided

3 large eggs, beaten

2 large carrots, diced

6 green onions, thinly sliced

2 tsp (6 g) minced garlic

½ tsp ground ginger

12 oz (340 g) fresh or frozen cauliflower rice

¼ cup (60 ml) coconut aminos, plus more as needed

½ tsp red pepper flakes

1 tbsp (15 ml) toasted sesame oil

1. Season the shrimp with the salt and black pepper. Heat 1 tablespoon (15 ml) of the avocado oil in a large skillet over medium-high heat. Add the shrimp and cook them for 1 to 2 minutes per side, or until they are just cooked through. Transfer the shrimp to a plate, and reduce the heat to medium.

2. Add the eggs and cook them for 1 to 2 minutes, until they are just set, breaking them into small pieces with a wooden spoon. Set the eggs aside with the shrimp.

3. Add the remaining 1 tablespoon (15 ml) of avocado oil to the skillet. Stir in the carrots. Cook the carrots for 3 to 4 minutes, or until they are just tender. Stir in the green onions, garlic and ginger.

4. Add the cauliflower rice, coconut aminos, red pepper flakes and sesame oil, and cook the mixture for 3 to 5 minutes, or until the cauliflower rice is just softened.

5. Stir the shrimp and eggs into the cauliflower rice and cook the fried rice for 1 minute, until it is warmed through. Serve the fried rice hot with more coconut aminos.

EASY BAKED CHICKEN RATATOUILLE

Ratatouille is a French vegetable stew full of roasted-vegetable flavor and fresh herbs. This one is done in the easiest way possible: It's baked in the oven all at once, with a balsamic herb "dressing" for an extra flavor punch and plenty of fresh chicken to make it a complete meal. This makes a great meal-prep dish that you can easily serve over gluten-free pasta or potatoes if you like.

YIELD: 6 SERVINGS

2 tbsp (30 ml) olive oil

1 medium eggplant, cut into bite-size pieces

2 medium zucchini, roughly chopped

1 cup (66 g) thinly sliced cremini mushrooms

½ medium white onion, diced

1 medium red bell pepper, diced

1 (15-oz [425-g]) can fire-roasted diced tomatoes, with liquid

2 lbs (907 g) boneless, skinless chicken breasts or thighs, cut into 1" (2.5-cm) pieces

3 tbsp (45 ml) balsamic vinegar

2 tbsp (18 g) finely chopped garlic

1 tsp Italian seasoning

½ tsp salt

½ tsp black pepper

1. Preheat the oven to 400°F (204°C). Grease a 9 x 13–inch (23 x 33–cm) glass baking dish with the oil, lightly coating the bottom and sides.

2. Add the eggplant, zucchini, mushrooms, onion, bell pepper, tomatoes, chicken, vinegar, garlic, Italian seasoning, salt and black pepper to the prepared baking dish. Toss the ingredients lightly with a large spoon to combine.

3. Bake the ratatouille for 45 minutes, or until the chicken is cooked through and the vegetables are tender.

4. Serve the ratatouille hot.

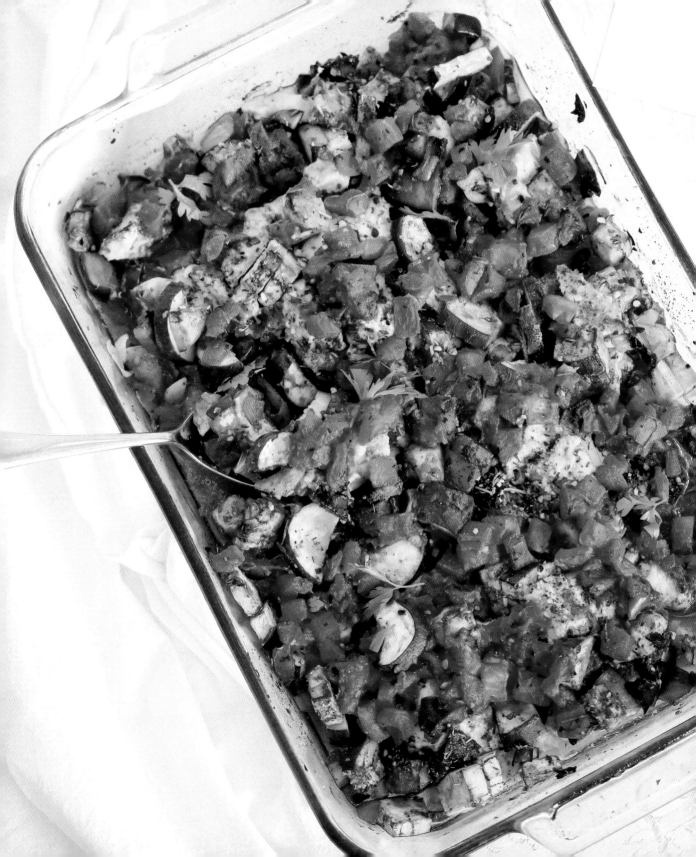

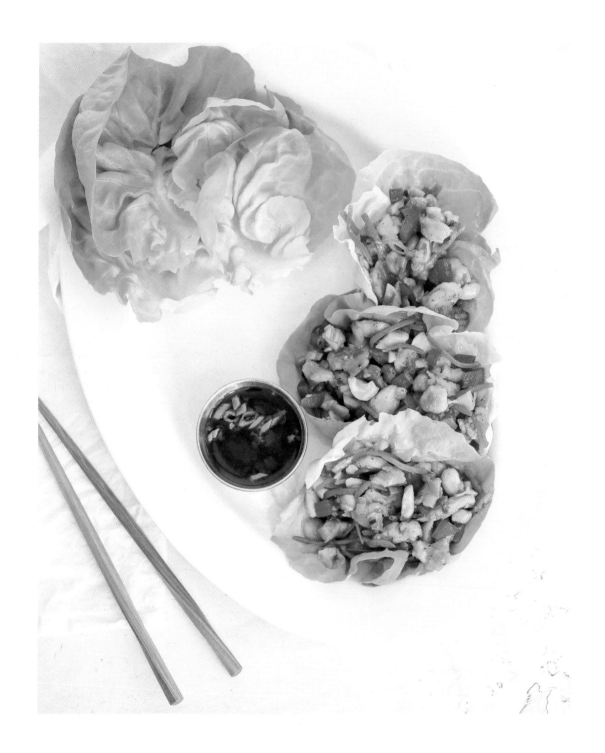

CASHEW CHICKEN LETTUCE WRAPS

Mouthwatering cashew chicken with tangy Asian sauce, tender veggies and toasted cashews are served lettuce wrap–style for the ultimate easy dish! In our house, we make the cashew chicken ahead of time and warm it before serving. It's just as tasty on a bed of cauliflower rice or salad.

YIELD: 8 LETTUCE WRAPS

SAUCE

½ cup (120 ml) coconut aminos, plus more as needed

3 tbsp (45 ml) rice vinegar

1 tbsp (15 ml) toasted sesame oil

1 (2" [5-cm]) piece fresh ginger, grated

2 tsp (6 g) minced garlic

½ tsp red pepper flakes

CASHEW CHICKEN

¾ cup (83 g) raw cashews, roughly chopped

2 tbsp (30 ml) avocado or coconut oil

2 lbs (908 g) boneless, skinless chicken thighs, cut into bite-size pieces

Salt, as needed

Black pepper, as needed

1 medium red bell pepper, diced

½ medium white onion, diced

½ cup (25 g) shredded carrots

½ cup (50 g) thinly sliced green onions

1 tsp minced garlic

2 tbsp (16 g) arrowroot flour plus 2 tbsp (30 ml) water

Leaves of 1 medium head butter lettuce

1. To make the sauce, whisk together the coconut aminos, vinegar, sesame oil, ginger, garlic and red pepper flakes in a small bowl until the sauce is smooth. Set the bowl aside.

2. To make the cashew chicken, toast the cashews in a large skillet over medium heat for 3 to 4 minutes, or until they are golden brown. Set the cashews aside. Add the avocado oil to the skillet and heat it over medium-high heat. Season the chicken with the salt and black pepper. Add the chicken to the skillet and cook it for 5 minutes, or until it is golden on all sides. Transfer the chicken to a plate, leaving the juices and oil in the skillet.

3. Add the bell pepper, onion and carrots to the skillet and cook them for 4 to 5 minutes, or until they are tender. Stir the chicken into the vegetable mixture. Add the green onions and garlic. Cook the mixture for 2 to 3 minutes, or until the chicken is warm and cooked through.

4. Stir in the cashews and sauce. In the same bowl used for the sauce, combine the arrowroot flour and water until the slurry is smooth. Stir the slurry into the cashew chicken mixture and cook it for 2 to 3 minutes to thicken the sauce.

5. Serve the cashew chicken scooped into the lettuce leaves to create wraps. Dip the wraps in additional coconut aminos.

PORK CHOPS WITH CINNAMON APPLES

These lightly crusted pork chops are a family favorite, but when they're served up with sautéed cinnamon apples? Then they are the best classic combination of sweet and savory that works every time. The sweetness of the cinnamon apples plays perfectly with the mild flavor of the pork, and the combination makes for the ideal bite. Serve this dish just like it's written or with some roasted green beans or a big green salad and enjoy!

YIELD: 4 SERVINGS

4 medium pork chops

2 tbsp (12 g) almond flour

½ tsp garlic powder

½ tsp dried rosemary

½ tsp dried sage

½ tsp salt

½ tsp black pepper

2 medium Pink Lady apples, cut into ⅛" (3-mm)-thick slices

½ tsp ground cinnamon

2 tbsp (30 g) ghee

1. Preheat the oven to 425°F (218°C). Lay the pork chops on a cutting board or a flat work surface covered with parchment paper. In a small bowl, combine the almond flour, garlic powder, rosemary, sage, salt and black pepper. Distribute the seasoning evenly among the pork chops, patting it onto both sides.

2. Place the apples in a medium bowl. Sprinkle them with the cinnamon. Use your hands to mix and coat them evenly.

3. Heat the ghee in a large ovenproof skillet over medium-high heat. Add the pork chops and cook them for 3 minutes on the first side and 2 minutes on the second side, or until each side is light golden brown. (Don't worry about cooking them through at this point.) Set the pork chops aside on a plate.

4. Add the apples to the hot skillet, and sauté them for about 2 minutes.

5. Add the pork chops back to the skillet, nestling them among the apples so that they touch the bottom of the skillet. Bake the pork chops and apples for 8 minutes, or until the pork chops' internal temperature is 145°F (63°C).

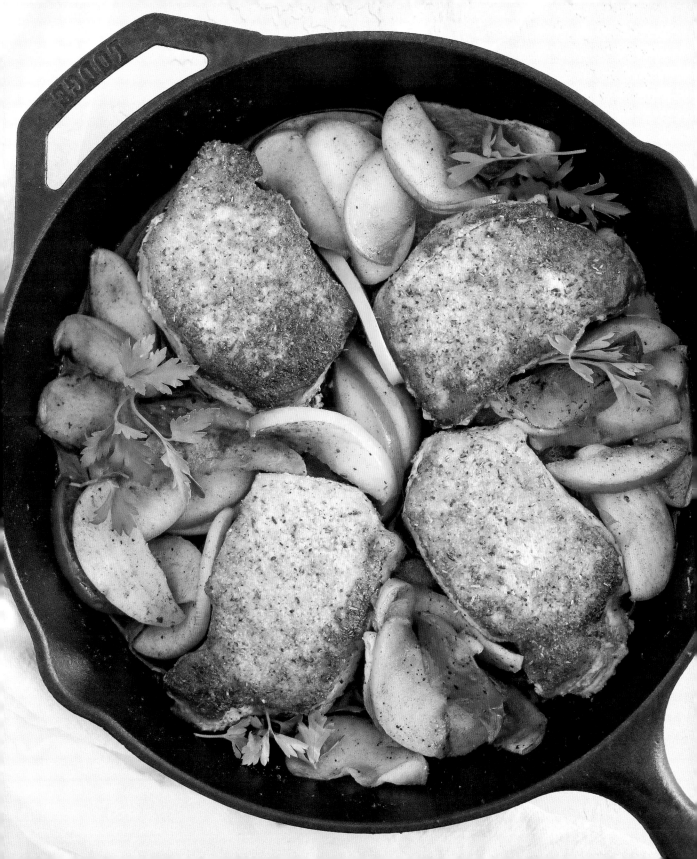

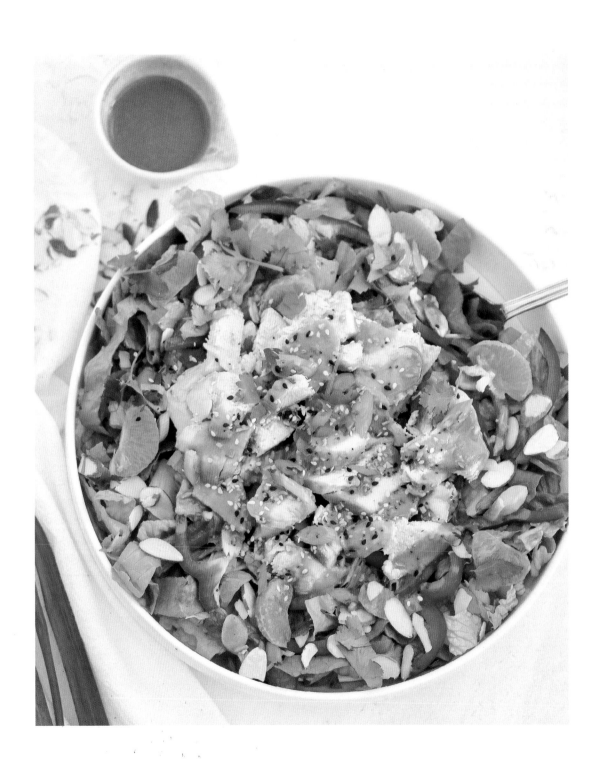

CHOPPED CHINESE CHICKEN SALAD WITH PEANUT-STYLE DRESSING

My secret to the easiest salad? Making it all in one bowl—including the dressing! Start by whisking up the dressing, then toss in the salad ingredients to lightly coat them. It works perfectly for this creamy, tangy Chinese chicken salad, which is one of our family favorites all year long.

YIELD: 4 SERVINGS

PEANUT-STYLE DRESSING

¼ cup (45 g) cashew butter

3 tbsp (45 ml) coconut aminos

2 tbsp (30 ml) rice vinegar

1 tbsp (15 ml) honey

1 tbsp (15 ml) toasted sesame oil

1 tsp minced garlic

1 (½" [13-mm]) piece fresh ginger, minced

SALAD

4 cups (300 g) roughly chopped romaine lettuce

3 cups (420 g) roughly chopped cooked boneless, skinless chicken breasts or thighs

½ medium red bell pepper, thinly sliced

½ cup (98 g) Mandarin orange slices

½ cup (55 g) sliced almonds

¼ cup (25 g) thinly sliced green onions

¼ cup (4 g) roughly chopped fresh cilantro

Toasted sesame seeds or bagel seasoning blend, as needed (optional)

1. To make the peanut-style dressing, vigorously whisk together the cashew butter, coconut aminos, vinegar, honey, oil, garlic and ginger in a large salad bowl until the dressing is smooth. Keep half of the dressing in the bowl, and transfer the other half to a small bowl. Set the small bowl of dressing aside.

2. To the dressing in the salad bowl, add the lettuce, chicken, bell pepper, Mandarin oranges, almonds, green onions and cilantro. Use tongs or two large forks to toss the ingredients until the salad is evenly coated with the dressing.

3. Serve the salad chilled with the remaining dressing and the sesame seeds (if using) on top.

NOTE: For a smooth dressing super quick, place all of the dressing ingredients in a small blender and pulse until the dressing is smooth. Add half of the dressing to the large salad bowl before tossing, and save the other half for drizzling.

BAKED SALMON AND ASPARAGUS IN PARCHMENT

Salmon en papillote, "salmon in paper," is the fancy French name for this dish. It's the ultimate one-dish meal: Fish and vegetables cooked in one pouch until they are tender. This method works with a variety of vegetables and flavor combinations, but this one with fresh garlic, lemon and asparagus is my hands-down favorite.

YIELD: 4 SERVINGS

40 asparagus spears

4 tbsp (60 ml) olive oil, divided

Salt, as needed

Black pepper, as needed

4 (6-oz [170-g]) skin-on salmon fillets

4 tsp (12 g) minced garlic

8 thin slices lemon

Roughly chopped fresh dill, as needed

1. Preheat the oven to 350°F (177°C). Fold 4 (12 x 18–inch [30 x 45–cm]) pieces of parchment paper in half down the middle, then open them back up.

2. Place 10 asparagus spears on one side of each piece of parchment paper. Drizzle them with ½ tablespoon (8 ml) of the oil and season them with salt and black pepper.

3. Top each serving of asparagus with 1 salmon fillet, 1 teaspoon of minced garlic and another ½ tablespoon (8 ml) of oil. Season the salmon with salt and black pepper, and then top each fillet with 2 slices of lemon.

4. Fold the parchment paper over the salmon and cinch the paper together by folding it over itself along the edges so the packet is tightly closed. Place the salmon packets on a large baking sheet.

5. Bake the packets for 20 minutes, or until the salmon is just cooked through and flakes easily with a fork. Garnish the salmon with the dill and serve the salmon and asparagus hot.

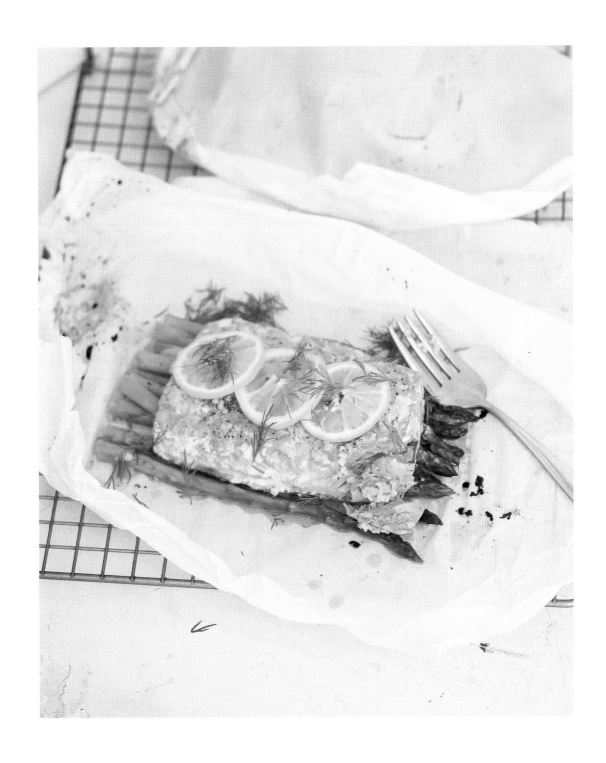

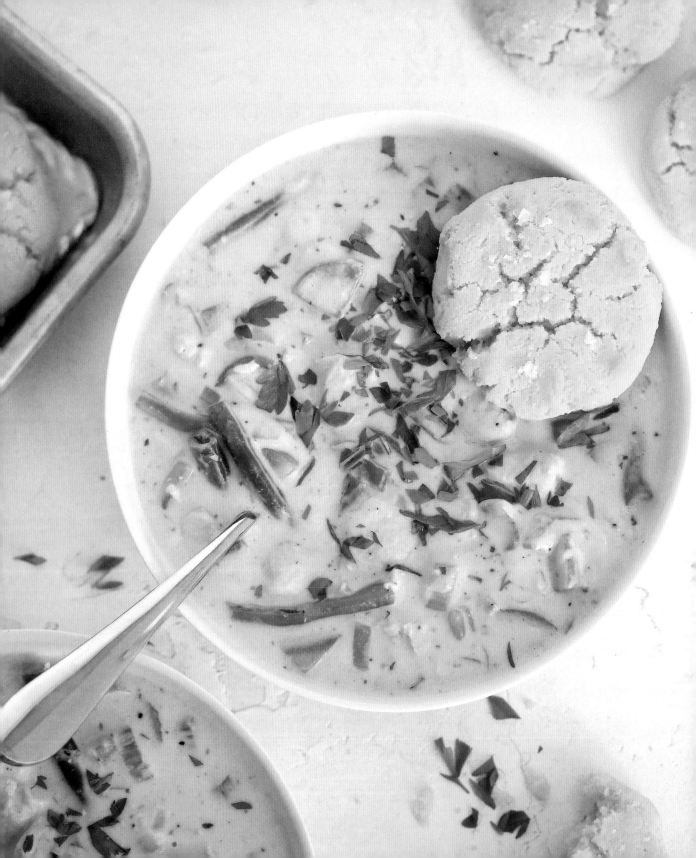

CHICKEN POT PIE CHOWDER

Chicken pot pie was one of my childhood cozy favorites—savory, rich and full of tender vegetables and juicy chicken. This chowder version takes all of that goodness and makes it Paleo friendly and super simple with a rich, creamy base and all of the flavor I love. Serve it with some warm One-Bowl Buttery Biscuits (page 115) to satisfy that crust craving.

YIELD: 6 SERVINGS

2 tbsp (30 g) grass-fed butter or ghee

3 large carrots, diced

3 medium ribs celery, diced

1 medium white or yellow onion, diced

2 tsp (6 g) minced garlic

1½ lbs (680 g) boneless, skinless chicken breasts

½ tsp dried rosemary

½ tsp dried sage

½ tsp dried oregano

½ tsp salt, plus more to taste

½ tsp black pepper, plus more to taste

4 cups (960 ml) chicken broth, divided

1 cup (240 ml) unsweetened coconut or almond milk

1 cup (111 g) raw cashews

1 cup (110 g) fresh green beans, cut to 2" (5-cm) pieces

Roughly chopped fresh parsley, as needed

1. Heat the butter in a large pot over medium-high heat. Add the carrots, celery, onion and garlic and sauté them for about 5 minutes, or until the vegetables are crisp-tender.

2. Add the chicken breasts to the pot. Add the rosemary, sage, oregano, salt, black pepper and 3 cups (720 ml) of the broth. Bring the mixture to a low boil, then reduce the heat to medium-low and bring the mixture to a simmer. Cook the mixture for about 20 minutes, or until the chicken's internal temperature is 165°F (74°C).

3. Remove the chicken from the pot and chop it into small pieces. Set the chicken aside. In a blender, combine the remaining 1 cup (240 ml) of broth, coconut milk and cashews. Blend until the ingredients are smooth to make cashew cream.

4. Stir the cashew cream, chicken and green beans into the chowder. Simmer the chowder for about 5 minutes, until the green beans are tender.

5. Season the chowder with additional salt and black pepper to taste. Garnish with the parsley and serve it hot.

TEX-MEX TACO SKILLET

All of your favorite taco flavors come together in one 15-minute skillet that's packed with veggies and loaded with classic taco toppings. Try this meal straight from the bowl, or wrap it up in a charred Paleo tortilla for something extra!

YIELD: 4 SERVINGS

TACO SEASONING

1 tbsp (11 g) nutritional yeast

1 tbsp (9 g) chili powder

1½ tsp (5 g) ground cumin

1 tsp garlic powder

1 tsp onion powder

½ tsp red pepper flakes

½ tsp dried oregano

½ tsp paprika

½ tsp salt

½ tsp black pepper

TACO SKILLET

1 tbsp (15 ml) avocado oil

2 lbs (907 g) ground beef

12 oz (340 g) fresh or frozen cauliflower rice

1 medium red onion, diced

1 medium green bell pepper, diced

1 (4-oz [113-g]) can diced green chiles, with liquid

1 (15-oz [425-g]) can fire-roasted diced tomatoes, with liquid

Spicy Ranch (page 16), as needed (optional)

Sliced limes, as needed (optional)

Guacamole, as needed (optional)

Chopped fresh cilantro, as needed (optional)

Hot sauce, as needed (optional)

1. To make the taco seasoning, combine the nutritional yeast, chili powder, cumin, garlic powder, onion powder, red pepper flakes, oregano, paprika, salt and black pepper in a small bowl.

2. To make the taco skillet, heat the oil in a large skillet over medium-high heat. Add the beef and 2 to 3 tablespoons (18 to 27 g) of the taco seasoning, depending on your spice preference. Cook the beef for 7 to 8 minutes, until it is crumbled and browned.

3. Stir in the cauliflower rice, onion and bell pepper. Cook the mixture for about 5 minutes, or until the vegetables are tender.

4. Add the green chiles and tomatoes, and stir to combine. Cook the mixture for 2 to 3 minutes, or until it is warmed through.

5. Place the taco mixture into bowls and top each serving with the Spicy Ranch (if using), lime wedges (if using), guacamole (if using), cilantro (if using) and hot sauce (if using).

NOTE: While the ingredients for the taco seasoning make just enough for a single batch of this recipe, you can make extra seasoning, transfer it to an airtight container and store it in a cool, dry place for up to 6 months.

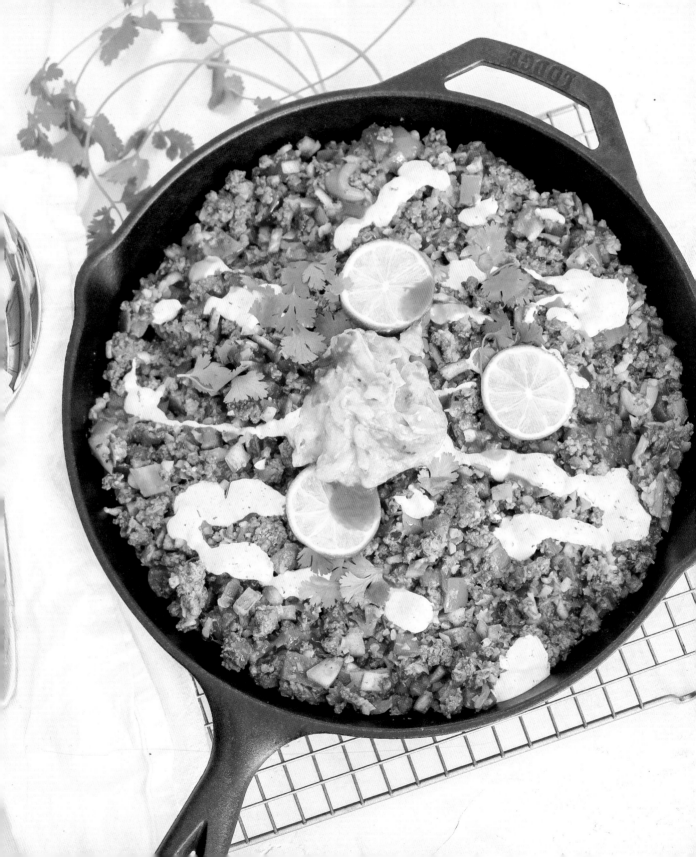

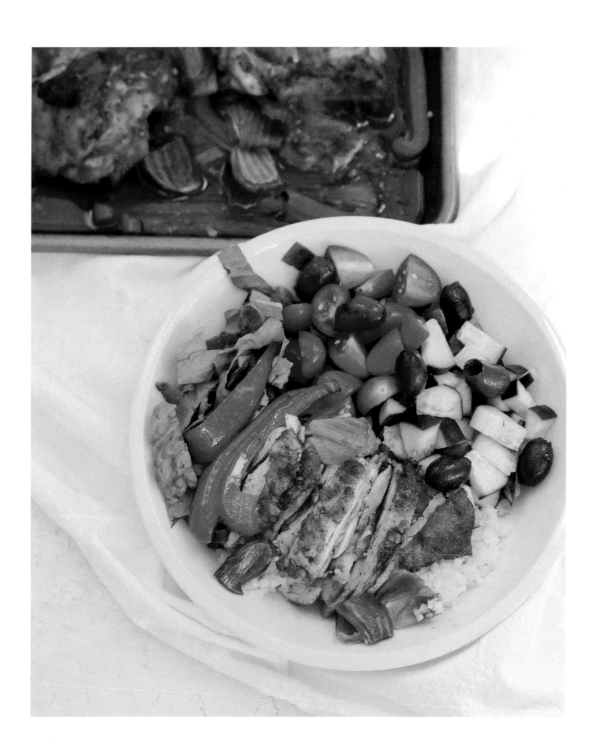

SHEET PAN CHICKEN SHAWARMA BOWLS

This well-marinated chicken shawarma will take you straight to the Mediterranean with a blend of warm spices mixed with fresh lemon and olive oil. While rotisserie-style chicken is typical for this dish, I roast it in the oven to keep it simple and serve it over fresh chilled vegetables. The result is a light-yet-satisfying meal that is bursting with unexpected flavors my family loves!

YIELD: 6 SERVINGS

Juice of 2 medium lemons, plus more as needed

⅓ cup (80 ml) olive oil, plus more as needed

6 cloves garlic, minced

2 tsp (5 g) black pepper, plus more as needed

2 tsp (6 g) ground cumin

2 tsp (6 g) paprika

1 tsp salt, plus more as needed

½ tsp ground turmeric

¼ tsp ground cinnamon

¼ tsp red pepper flakes, or more as needed

6 medium bone-in or boneless chicken thighs

1 large red onion, cut into 1" (2.5-cm) pieces

1 large red bell pepper, thinly sliced

3 cups (340 g) cauliflower rice

3 cups (225 g) finely chopped romaine lettuce

1½ cups (202 g) pitted Kalamata olives

1½ cups (224 g) cherry tomatoes, quartered

1½ cups (200 g) diced cucumber

1. In a large bowl, whisk together the lemon juice, oil, garlic, black pepper, cumin, paprika, salt, turmeric, cinnamon and red pepper flakes until the mixture is smooth. Add the chicken to the marinade and cover the bowl with a lid or foil. Refrigerate the chicken and allow the chicken to marinate for at least 30 minutes, or up to overnight.

2. Preheat the oven to 425°F (218°C). Arrange the chicken in a single layer on a large rimmed baking sheet. Nestle the onion and bell pepper around the chicken, and drizzle any remaining marinade over the top of the ingredients.

3. Roast the chicken and vegetables for 35 to 40 minutes, or until the chicken's internal temperature is 165°F (74°C).

4. Prepare the bowls by dividing the cauliflower rice, lettuce, olives, tomatoes and cucumber evenly among six bowls. Drizzle the vegetables with additional oil, season them with additional salt and black pepper and drizzle them with additional lemon juice. Top the vegetables with the cooked chicken and vegetables and serve.

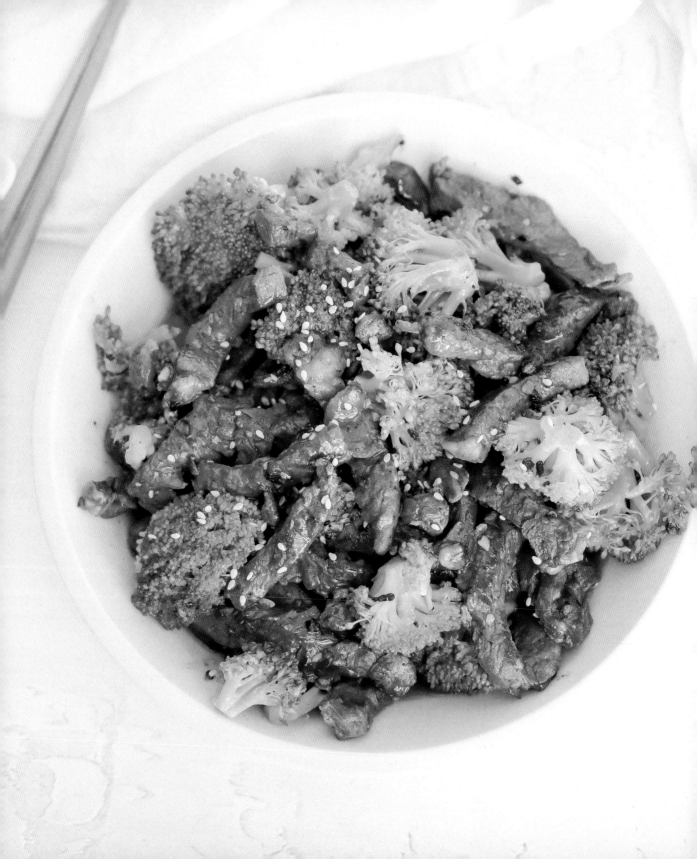

Five-Ingredient Dinners

Nothing says simplicity in the kitchen like a five-ingredient meal. However, when you love flavor like I do, keeping it simple can't mean keeping it boring. In this chapter, I take five easy main ingredients and transform them into satisfying, savory dishes the whole family will love. The only ingredients not counted toward the five are the cooking fat, salt and black pepper. I've listed some optional garnishes as well to finish things off—but know that even with the basic ingredients listed, you're going to be all set with a delicious meal created from pantry basics!

SPAGHETTI SQUASH WITH MEAT SAUCE

Classic, never-gets-old spaghetti and meat sauce gets a Paleo makeover with roasted spaghetti squash. Serve it with a hearty semi-homemade meat sauce for the simplest dinner that comes together quick and never disappoints!

YIELD: 2 TO 4 SERVINGS

1 medium spaghetti squash

2 tbsp (30 ml) olive oil, divided

1 lb (454 g) ground beef

½ medium white onion, diced

1 tbsp (9 g) minced garlic

1 (32-oz [946-ml]) jar marinara sauce

Red pepper flakes, as needed (optional)

Roughly chopped fresh basil, as needed (optional)

1. Preheat the oven to 375°F (191°C). Line a large baking sheet with parchment paper and set it aside. Slice the spaghetti squash in half and drizzle each half lightly with a ½ tablespoon (7 ml) of the oil, then place the squash cut side down on the prepared baking sheet.

2. Roast the squash for 45 minutes, or until it is fork-tender.

3. Heat the remaining tablespoon (15 ml) of oil in a large skillet over medium-high heat. Add the beef and cook it for about 5 minutes, until it is crumbly and browned. Add the onion and garlic and cook the mixture for 3 to 4 minutes, until the onion is translucent. Stir in the marinara sauce and simmer until the sauce is warmed through.

4. Scoop the spaghetti squash strands out into four bowls, or serve the squash in the skin for a larger double portion. Spoon the meat sauce over the top of the squash, and garnish it with the red pepper flakes (if using) and basil (if using).

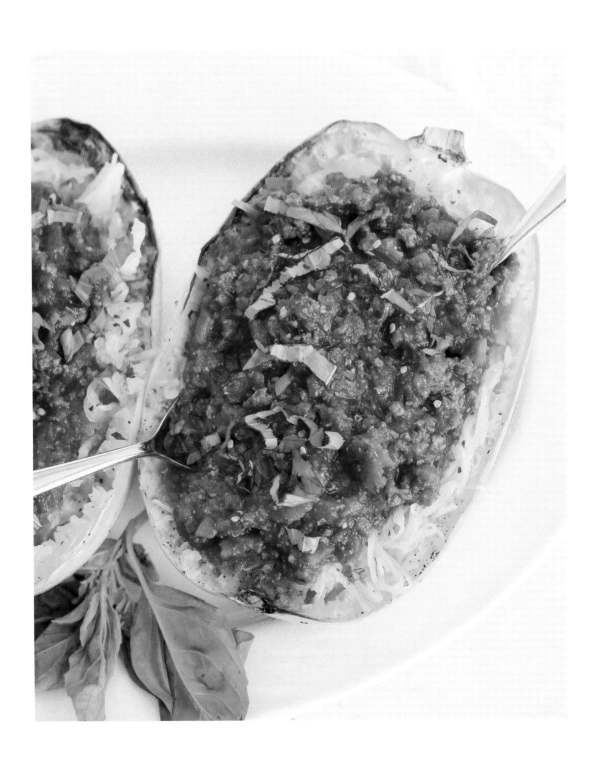

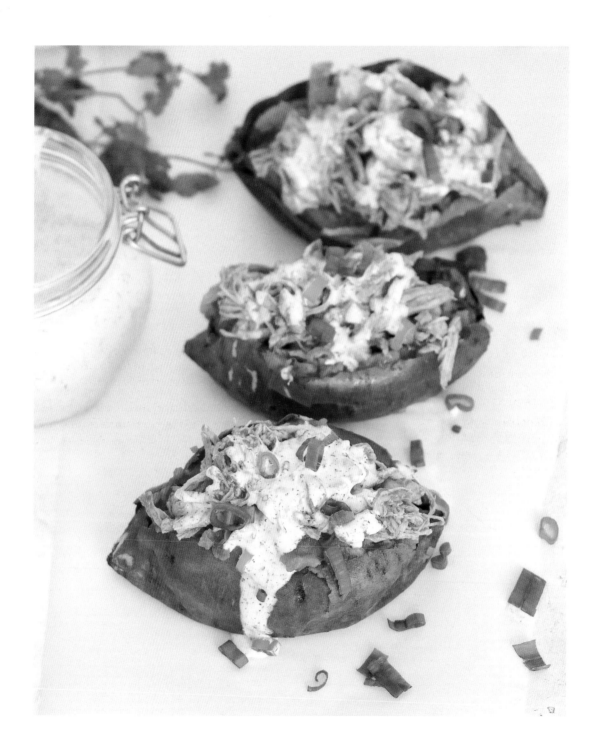

BUFFALO CHICKEN–STUFFED SWEET POTATOES

The classic combination of sweet and savory is taken to the next level with this easy stuffed sweet potato meal. The potatoes are roasted until they are soft and extra sweet, while the chicken is simmered in a spicy Buffalo-style sauce, taken down just a notch with creamy coconut milk—although you won't be tasting the coconut in this dish. Top the potatoes with cool, creamy ranch to round it out, and dig in!

YIELD: 4 SERVINGS

4 medium sweet potatoes

2 cups (250 g) shredded cooked chicken breast

¼ to ⅓ cup (60 to 80 ml) hot sauce

¼ cup (60 ml) coconut milk

Quick Homemade Ranch (page 123) or store-bought Paleo ranch dressing, as needed

Roughly chopped fresh cilantro, as needed (optional)

Thinly sliced green onions, as needed (optional)

1. Preheat the oven to 400°F (204°C). Scrub the sweet potatoes and poke a few small holes in them with a fork. Arrange them on a large baking sheet. Bake the sweet potatoes for 45 minutes, or until they are soft on the inside.

2. In a medium saucepan over medium heat, combine the chicken, hot sauce and coconut milk. Simmer the mixture for 10 minutes to allow the flavors to combine and the sauce to slightly thicken.

3. Slice the cooked sweet potatoes down the middle to open them up. Scoop the Buffalo chicken into the sweet potatoes and top each serving with the Quick Homemade Ranch, cilantro (if using) and green onions (if using). Serve the potatoes warm.

ITALIAN SAUSAGE AND PEPPERS SKILLET

I learned how to make this dish in a high school cooking class, and I have made it simpler over the years as life has gotten busier. The flavors are still incredible, and it tastes like pure Italian comfort food. I once served this on toasted ciabatta buns, but now I get just as much joy from eating it straight out of the bowl!

YIELD: 4 SERVINGS

1 tbsp (15 ml) olive oil

1 lb (454 g) sweet, mild or hot Italian sausages

2 medium red or green bell peppers, sliced into 2" to 3" (5- to 7.5-cm) strips

1 medium white or yellow onion, sliced into ⅛" (3-mm)-thick strips

2 tsp (6 g) minced garlic

1½ cups (360 ml) marinara sauce

Roughly chopped fresh parsley, as needed (optional)

Red pepper flakes, as needed (optional)

1. Heat the oil in a large skillet over medium-high heat. Add the sausages and cook them for 7 to 10 minutes, until they are browned on all sides and cooked through in the center. Transfer the sausages to a plate and set the plate aside.

2. Add the bell peppers, onion and garlic to the skillet, and sauté the vegetables for about 5 minutes, until they are crisp-tender. Stir in the marinara sauce and reduce the heat to medium-low.

3. Slice the sausages into three pieces each, and then nestle them among the vegetables in the skillet. Cook the mixture until the sausages are warmed through.

4. Garnish the sausages and peppers with the parsley (if using) and red pepper flakes (if using), then serve.

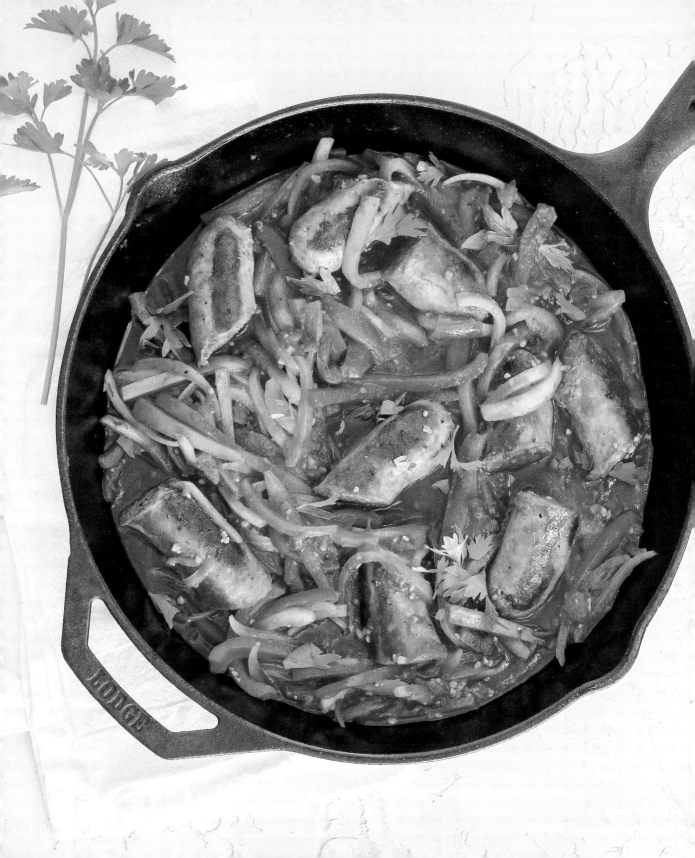

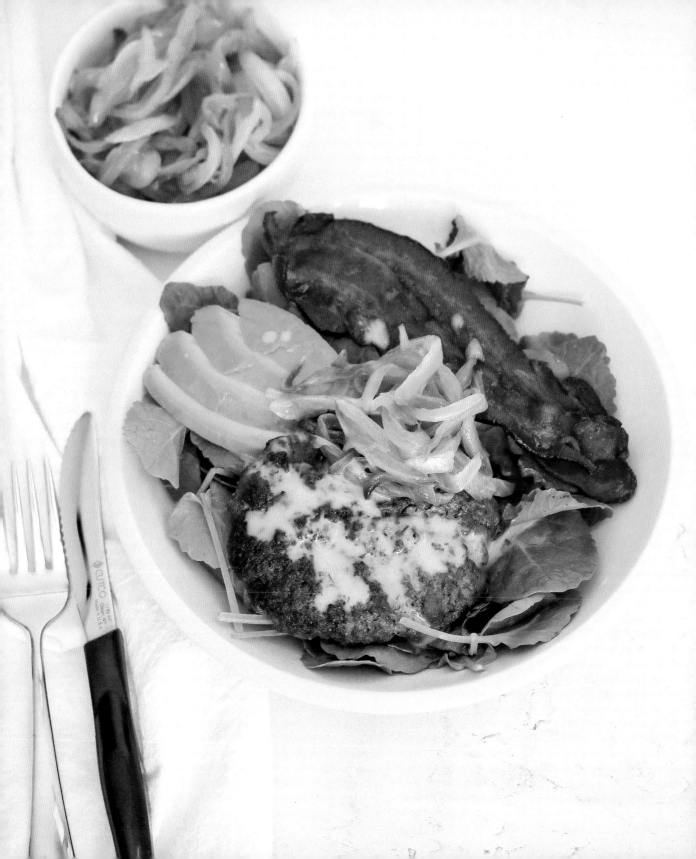

ABC BURGER BOWLS

ABC, these are easy as 1, 2, 3—and also my favorite burger! Avocado, bacon and caramelized onion makes for the best kind of ABCs in my book. The flavors here are big, but the dish is simple. Make extra bacon and onions ahead of time, and keep them on hand for adding to salads, breakfasts and more.

YIELD: 4 SERVINGS

BOWLS

8 slices of bacon

4 cups (120 g) baby spinach or baby kale

1 large avocado, quartered

Quick Homemade Ranch (page 123), Paleo barbecue sauce or condiments of choice, as needed (optional)

CARAMELIZED ONIONS

½ tbsp (8 ml) avocado oil

1 medium white or yellow onion, thinly sliced

Pinch of salt

BURGERS

1 lb (454 g) ground beef

2 tbsp (30 ml) avocado oil

Salt, as needed

Black pepper, as needed

1. To begin preparing the bowls, line a large rimmed baking sheet with parchment paper, and arrange the bacon on the baking sheet in a single layer. Transfer the baking sheet to a cold oven, then set the temperature to 400°F (204°C). Bake the bacon for 18 to 22 minutes total (including the preheating time), until it is crispy. Set the bacon aside.

2. To make the caramelized onions, heat the oil in a medium skillet over medium-low heat. Add the onion in a single layer. Cook the onion for 10 minutes, stirring occasionally to brown it evenly. Add the salt, stir the onion and cook for 15 to 20 minutes, or until the onion is caramelized. Don't stir the onion too often, as it needs to have a chance to brown.

3. To make the burgers, divide the beef into four ¼-inch (6-mm)-thick patties. Handle the meat as little as possible, just enough to flatten and shape the patties. Heat the oil in a large cast-iron skillet over medium-high heat. Season the burgers generously with the salt and black pepper on each side just before adding them to the skillet. Add the burgers to the skillet and cook them for 2 to 3 minutes per side, or until they are browned. Transfer them to a plate to rest until you are ready to serve.

4. To finish preparing the bowls, divide the spinach among four bowls. Layer the spinach with a burger patty, one-quarter of the avocado, 2 slices of bacon and a scoop of the caramelized onion. Garnish each serving with the Quick Homemade Ranch (if using).

BACON-WRAPPED CHICKEN AND GREEN BEANS

Anything wrapped in bacon is immediately better, and this juicy rubbed chicken breast is no exception! The spice rub for this dish is the perfect blend of sweet and savory and goes perfectly with smoky bacon. Roast the bacon-wrapped chicken on a sheet pan with tender-crisp green beans for a complete dish in no time.

YIELD: 4 SERVINGS

4 medium boneless, skinless chicken breasts

¼ cup (48 g) coconut sugar

1 tsp garlic powder

½ tsp salt, plus more as needed

½ tsp black pepper, plus more as needed

8 slices of bacon

12 to 16 oz (340 to 454 g) trimmed fresh green beans

Avocado or olive oil spray

1. Preheat the oven to 400°F (204°C). Place the chicken breasts on a cutting board or work surface covered with parchment paper. In a small bowl, combine the sugar, garlic powder, salt and black pepper.

2. Rub half of the seasoning mixture on the chicken breasts, coating both sides. Wrap each chicken breast with 2 slices of bacon, keeping the seams where the ends of the bacon slices meet at the bottom of the chicken breast. Arrange the bacon-wrapped chicken breasts on a large baking sheet. Sprinkle the remaining seasoning mixture over the top of the chicken.

3. Add the green beans to the baking sheet, nestling among the chicken breasts. Lightly spray the green beans with the avocado oil spray, and then season them with additional salt and black pepper.

4. Bake the chicken and green beans for 30 minutes, or until the chicken's internal temperature reaches 165°F (74°C). Increase the oven temperature to broil and cook the chicken and green beans for about 2 minutes to crisp the bacon, watching it closely so it doesn't burn.

5. Serve the chicken and green beans hot.

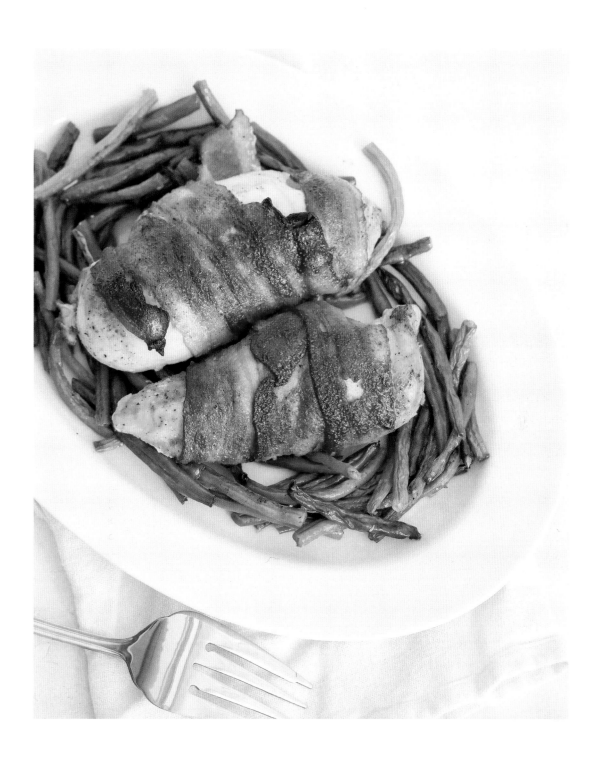

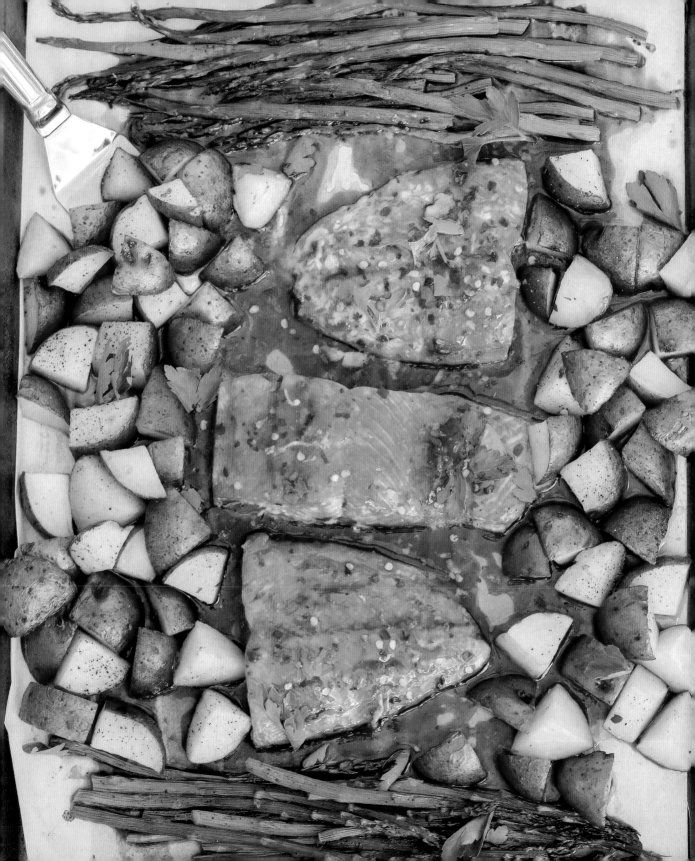

HONEY-GLAZED SALMON DINNER

All of dinner done in 30 minutes, with just one sheet pan to clean up? I'm all about it! This dish is the perfect pairing of salmon, potatoes and vegetables, with a honey glaze over the top that's to die for. Enjoy this on the busiest of weeknights or on a weekend date night.

YIELD: 3 SERVINGS

2 tbsp (30 ml) coconut aminos

2 tbsp (30 ml) honey

3 tbsp (45 ml) olive oil, divided

8 small to medium red potatoes, quartered

Salt, as needed

Black pepper, as needed

3 (6-oz [170-g]) skin-on salmon fillets

30 thin asparagus spears

Red pepper flakes, as needed (optional)

Finely chopped fresh parsley, as needed (optional)

1. Preheat the oven to 400°F (204°C). Line a large rimmed baking sheet with parchment paper. In a small bowl, whisk together the coconut aminos, honey and 2 tablespoons (30 ml) of the oil. Set the honey glaze aside.

2. Arrange the potatoes on the baking sheet in a single layer. Drizzle them with the remaining 1 tablespoon (15 ml) of oil and season them with salt and black pepper. Bake the potatoes for 20 minutes.

3. Remove the baking sheet from the oven, and use a spatula to scoot the potatoes to the edges of the baking sheet. Arrange the salmon fillets and asparagus spears in the center of the baking sheet and season them with salt and black pepper. Pour the honey glaze over the top of the salmon fillets.

4. Bake the mixture for 10 minutes, or until the salmon is just cooked through. Season the entire dish with red pepper flakes (if using) and fresh parsley (if using), and serve hot.

QUICK BROCCOLI AND BEEF STIR-FRY

In this recipe, five simple ingredients are put to work to re-create the classic Chinese broccoli and beef dish that I grew up loving almost as much as egg rolls. This Paleo version is soy-free and truly tastes like the real deal—or better! The marinade is delicious and does its job quickly, so this meal comes together fast.

YIELD: 4 SERVINGS

BROCCOLI AND BEEF STIR-FRY

2 tbsp (30 ml) coconut aminos

1 tbsp (15 ml) toasted sesame oil

½ tsp salt

¼ tsp black pepper or red pepper flakes

1 lb (454 g) beef, sliced ¼" (6 mm) thick (see Note)

4 cups (700 g) medium broccoli florets

1 tbsp (15 ml) avocado oil

1 tsp minced garlic

Toasted sesame seeds, as needed (optional)

STIR-FRY SAUCE

3 tbsp (45 ml) coconut aminos

1 tbsp (15 ml) toasted sesame oil

¼ tsp red pepper flakes

1. To make the broccoli and beef stir-fry, whisk together the coconut aminos, sesame oil, salt and black pepper in a large, shallow dish. Add the beef and cover the dish with its lid or some foil, and transfer it to the refrigerator to marinate for at least 15 minutes or up to 1 hour.

2. Steam the broccoli by placing the florets in a large skillet containing ½ to 1 inch (13 mm to 2.5 cm) of water. Heat the skillet over medium-high heat until the water comes to a low boil. Cover the skillet with a lid and cook the broccoli for 3 to 4 minutes, until it turns bright green and is crisp-tender. Drain the water and keep the broccoli covered until you are ready to serve.

3. Heat the avocado oil in a large skillet or wok over medium-high heat. Add the garlic and marinated beef, cooking the beef in batches so the skillet isn't overcrowded for about 2 minutes per side, or until the beef is crisp and browned.

4. To make the stir-fry sauce, whisk together the coconut aminos, sesame oil and red pepper flakes in a small bowl. Add the stir-fry sauce to the skillet and cook the beef and sauce for about 1 minute to warm the dish through. Stir in the broccoli, tossing to coat it with the sauce. Garnish the stir-fry with the sesame seeds (if using). Serve the stir-fry hot.

NOTE: Just about any tender cut of beef will work for this. My family likes rib eye, sirloin, skirt steak or flank steak.

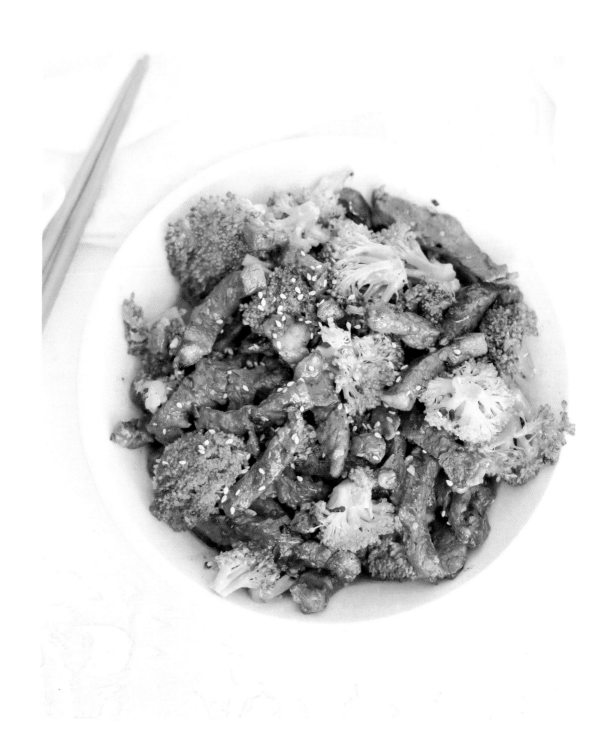

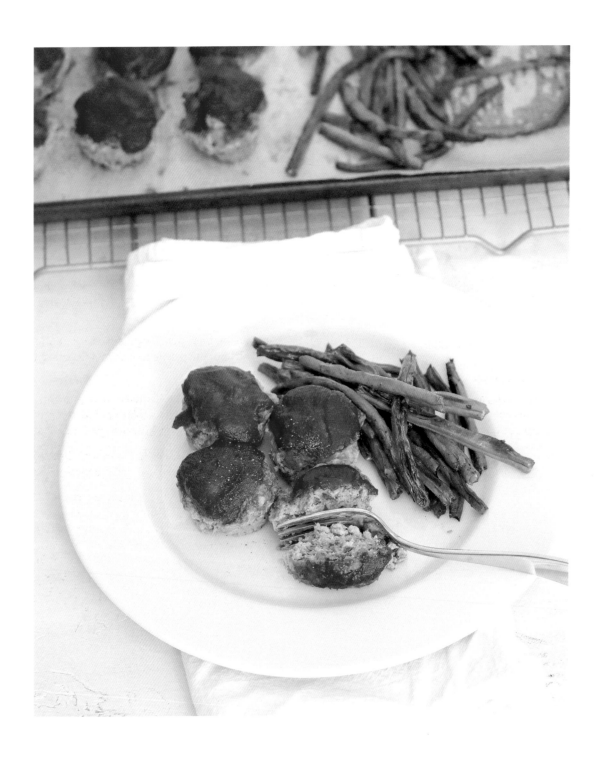

MEATLOAF MUFFINS WITH ROASTED GREEN BEANS

Two dishes, one meal—all cooked together at the same time and temperature. These meatloaf muffins are the perfect protein-packed bite, topped with your choice of Paleo-friendly ketchup or pizza sauce for an easy dinner option. Fill your second dish with green beans that roast to tender perfection and make the perfect side. Dinner is done, and the whole family is guaranteed to love it!

YIELD: 4 SERVINGS

2 lbs (907 g) ground beef

1 cup (96 g) almond flour

2 large eggs

1 tsp salt, plus more as needed

1 tsp black pepper, plus more as needed

1 cup (240 ml) Paleo ketchup or pizza sauce, divided

1 lb (454 g) trimmed fresh green beans

1 tbsp (15 ml) olive oil

1   Preheat the oven to 350°F (177°C). Line a 12-well muffin pan with parchment paper or silicone liners. Line a large baking sheet with parchment paper.

2   In a large bowl, combine the beef, flour, eggs, salt, black pepper and ½ cup (120 ml) of the ketchup with a large fork or your fingers until the ingredients are just mixed.

3   Divide the mixture evenly between the 12 muffin wells, pressing down on the mixture in each well to fill it completely. Top the meatloaf muffins with the remaining ½ cup (120 ml) of ketchup or pizza sauce.

4   Arrange the green beans on the prepared baking sheet. Drizzle them with the oil and season them with additional salt and black pepper.

5   Transfer both the muffin pan and baking sheet to the oven, and bake the meatloaf muffins and green beans for 25 to 30 minutes, or until the meatloaf muffins' internal temperature reaches 160°F (71°C) and the green beans are tender. Serve the meatloaf muffins and green beans warm.

SHRIMP TACO BOWLS WITH AVOCADO-LIME SLAW

Ready to take on taco night Paleo style with just five ingredients? This quick and easy dish is packed with charred taco flavor and made extra fresh and light with a simple slaw dressed with a creamy avocado-lime dressing. Make double the dressing and save it for dressing any salad or bowl throughout the week—it's so good, you'll want more!

YIELD: 4 SERVINGS

½ medium avocado

Juice of 2 medium limes

3 tbsp (45 ml) avocado oil, divided

1 lb (454 g) coleslaw cabbage mix

Salt, as needed

Black pepper, as needed

1 lb (454 g) fresh or thawed frozen shrimp, peeled and deveined

2 tsp (6 g) taco seasoning (see Note)

Finely chopped fresh cilantro, as needed (optional)

Hot sauce, as needed (optional)

Lime wedges, as needed (optional)

1. In a small blender, combine the avocado, lime juice and 2 tablespoons (30 ml) of the oil and blend until the ingredients are smooth. Transfer the dressing to a large bowl and add the coleslaw cabbage mix. Season the slaw with salt and black pepper and stir to combine the ingredients. Cover the bowl and refrigerate the slaw while you prepare the shrimp.

2. Season both sides of the shrimp with the taco seasoning. Heat the remaining 1 tablespoon (15 ml) of oil in a large skillet over medium-high heat. Add the shrimp and cook them for 1 to 2 minutes per side, or until they are browned and just cooked through.

3. Serve the avocado-lime slaw topped with the shrimp, cilantro (if using), hot sauce (if using) and lime wedges (if using).

NOTE: Try my Taco Seasoning recipe on page 54 or use a store-bought taco seasoning.

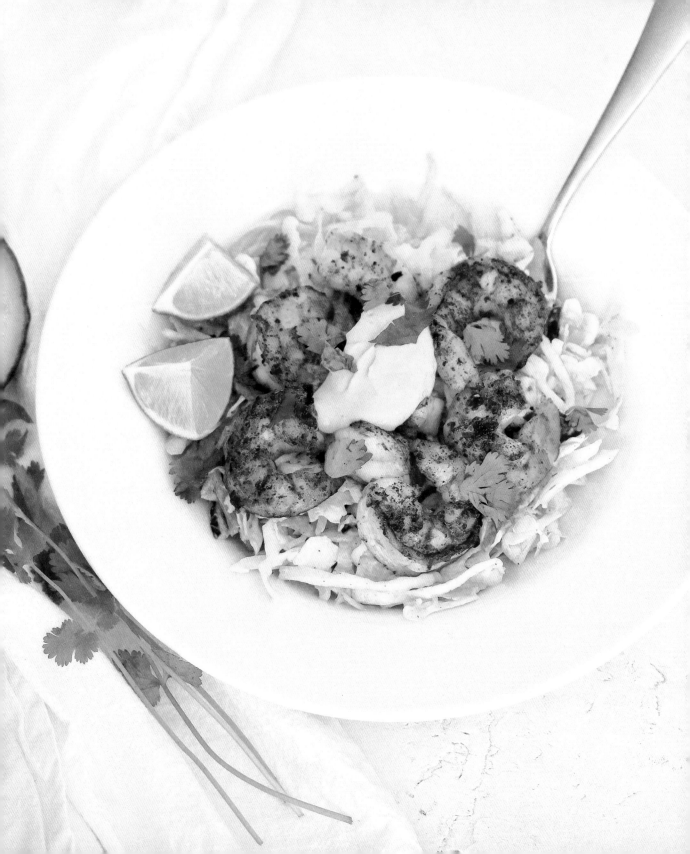

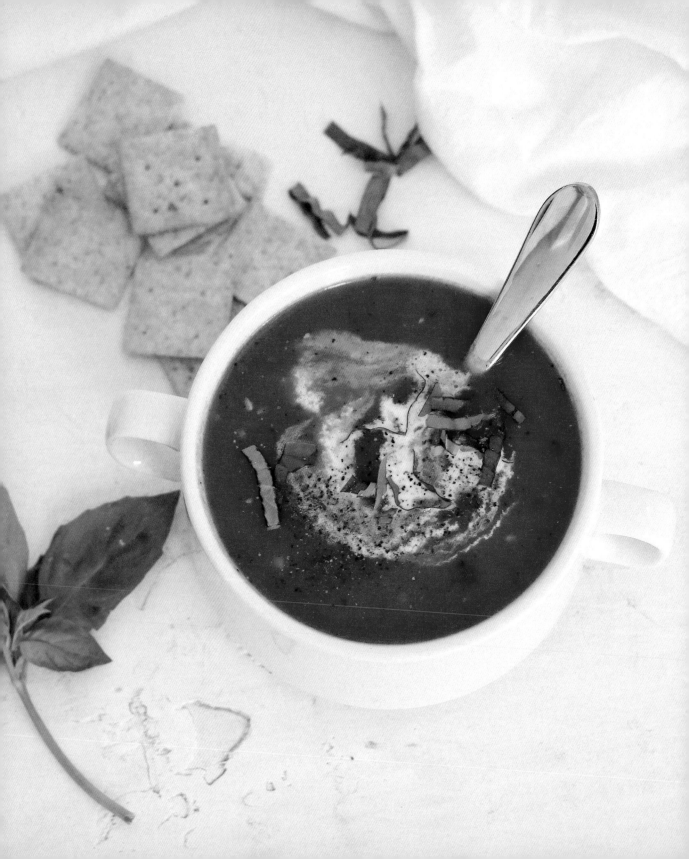

CREAMY TOMATO-BASIL BLENDER SOUP

This 10-minute soup is a classic favorite that's so simple to make. Using canned fire-roasted tomatoes makes it easy but also adds a great depth of flavor that will make the soup taste like it simmered for hours. Toasted garlic and fresh basil bring this soup to the next level— the perfect fresh and cozy bowl.

YIELD: 4 SERVINGS

2 (15-oz [425-g]) cans fire-roasted diced tomatoes, with liquid

1 cup (240 ml) chicken broth

1 tbsp (15 ml) olive oil

2 tsp (6 g) minced garlic

¼ cup (60 ml) coconut milk

¼ cup (15 g) finely chopped fresh basil, plus more as needed

Salt, as needed

Black pepper, as needed

1. In a blender, combine the tomatoes and broth and blend until the ingredients are smooth.

2. Heat the oil in a large pot over medium heat. Add the garlic and sauté it for 2 to 3 minutes, until it is golden and fragrant.

3. Stir in the tomato mixture, coconut milk and basil. Bring the soup to a simmer and cook it for about 5 minutes, until it is warmed through.

4. Season the soup with salt and black pepper. Garnish the soup with additional basil and serve it hot.

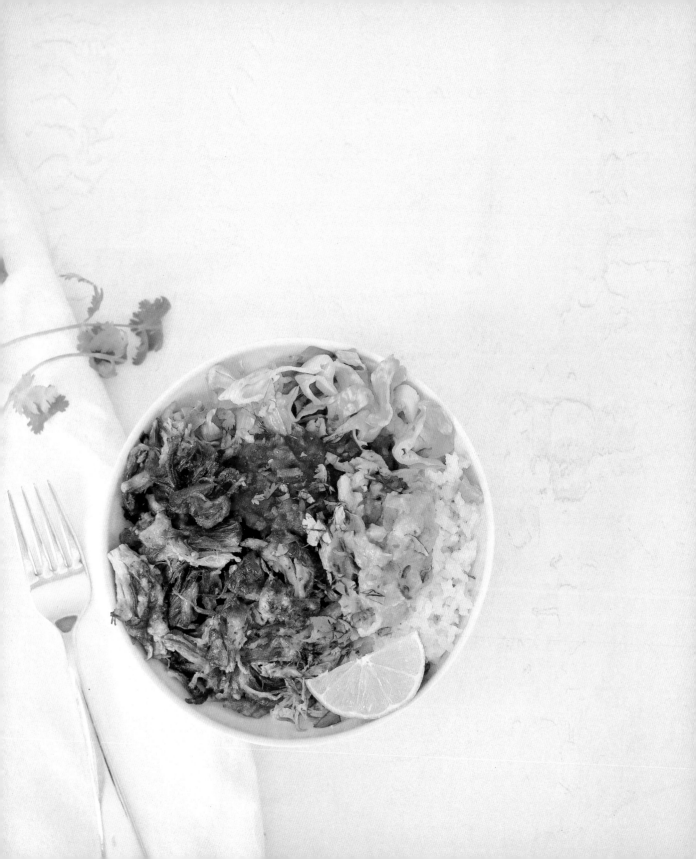

Fast and Slow Dinners

The Instant Pot pressure cooker and the slow cooker are two of my favorite kitchen tools, and I use them on a regular basis. Each appliance yields extra flavorful, perfectly cooked food that requires very little hands-on time. The difference is that the slow cooker requires some planning ahead (which can be great if you know you have a busy day at work and want dinner done when you get home), while the Instant Pot can give you the same results yet so much faster and is a great option for when you didn't plan a thing—which is me most days!

In this chapter, I give you delicious weeknight dinner recipes that can be done either way: over time in the slow cooker or quickly in the Instant Pot. So whether you're a super planner or more of a "What sounds good tonight?" kind of cook, you'll be set up for a tasty and time-saving dinnertime success.

SALSA VERDE FLANK STEAK TACOS

Taco night is a favorite around here because it's so easy, and everyone is left full and happy! Whip up this easy salsa verde flank steak, and serve it up however you like: over a big salad, in tortillas or even mixed into a scramble for breakfast the next day. The salsa verde adds a light, mild heat with fresh flavor that goes well with the tender, juicy steak—it truly melts in your mouth.

YIELD: 8 TACOS

1½ lbs (680 g) flank steak

Salt, as needed

Black pepper, as needed

1 tbsp (15 ml) avocado oil

1 cup (240 ml) salsa verde

8 (6" [15-cm]) Paleo tortillas

Guacamole, as needed (optional)

Roughly chopped fresh cilantro, as needed (optional)

Hot sauce, as needed (optional)

Diced red onion, as needed (optional)

INSTANT POT

1. Lay the flank steak on a large cutting board or a flat work surface that's been covered with parchment paper. Cut the steak into smaller pieces that will fit in the surface area of the bottom of the Instant Pot. Season each side of the meat generously with the salt and black pepper.

2. Set the Instant Pot to Sauté mode and add the oil. Once the oil is hot, add the steak in batches so that the pieces don't overlap. Sear the steak pieces for 3 to 4 minutes per side, until they are browned. Press Cancel to turn off the heat. Place all of the meat and the salsa verde in the pot.

3. Secure the lid on the Instant Pot in the locked position, and set the vent to sealing. Set the Instant Pot to Pressure Cook and cook the steak at high pressure for 45 minutes.

4. Once the Instant Pot is finished, manually release the steam by carefully moving the vent to the venting position until the valve has dropped. Remove the lid, and use two forks to shred the steak.

5. Warm the tortillas over a low open flame on a gas stove or toast them in a medium skillet over medium-low heat until they are lightly charred. Fill the tortillas with the flank steak and top the tacos with the guacamole (if using), cilantro (if using), hot sauce (if using) and red onion (if using).

(continued)

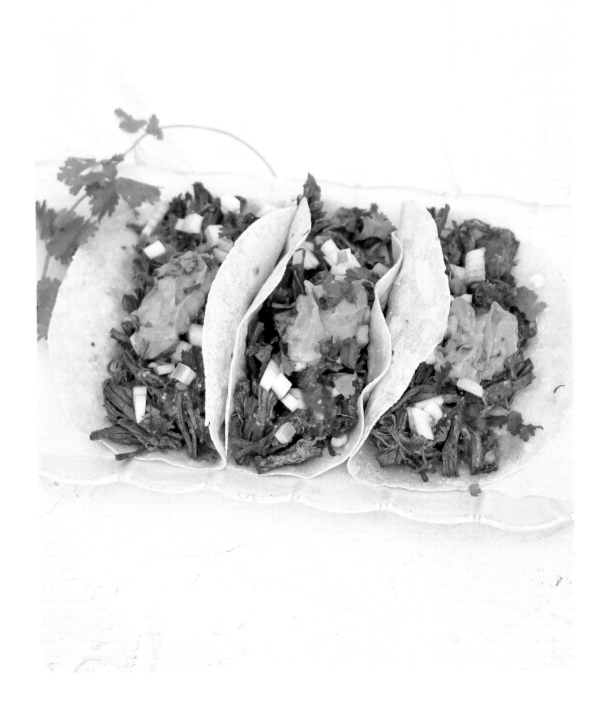

SALSA VERDE FLANK STEAK TACOS (CONT.)

SLOW COOKER

1. Lay the flank steak out on a large cutting board or a flat work surface that's been covered with parchment paper. Cut the steak into smaller pieces that are a maximum of 5 to 6 inches (13 to 15 cm) long. Season each side of the meat generously with the salt and black pepper.

2. Heat the oil in a large skillet over medium-high heat. Add the steak in batches so that the pieces don't overlap. Sear the steak pieces for 3 to 4 minutes per side, until they are browned.

3. Transfer the steak pieces to the slow cooker and add the salsa verde. Cover the slow cooker with its lid. Cook the steak on low for 6 hours, or until the meat is tender enough to shred. Shred the meat with two forks.

4. Warm the tortillas over a low open flame on a gas stove or toast them in a medium skillet over medium-low until they are lightly charred. Fill the tortillas with the flank steak and top the tacos with the guacamole (if using), cilantro (if using), hot sauce (if using) and red onion (if using).

CRISPY CARNITAS BURRITO BOWLS

Mouthwatering citrus carnitas are pressure- or slow-cooked to perfection then broiled until crispy and delicious. Serve this dish burrito bowl–style for an easy dinner that everyone can customize to their liking. I take mine extra crispy, with double guac!

YIELD: 8 SERVINGS

4 lbs (1.8 kg) boneless pork shoulder, cut into 3" (7.5-cm) cubes

2 cups (480 ml) chicken broth

Juice of 1 medium orange

Juice of 3 medium limes

2 tsp (6 g) ground cumin

2 tsp (10 g) salt

1 tsp black pepper

1 tsp dried oregano

2 tbsp (30 ml) avocado oil

8 cups (906 g) steamed cauliflower rice, divided

4 cups (300 g) finely chopped romaine lettuce, divided

Salsa, as needed (optional)

Guacamole, as needed (optional)

Roughly chopped fresh cilantro, as needed (optional)

Fresh lime juice, as needed (optional)

INSTANT POT

1. Add the pork to the Instant Pot and top the pork with the broth, orange juice, lime juice, cumin, salt, black pepper and oregano. Stir to combine the ingredients.

2. Secure the lid on the Instant Pot in the locked position, and set the vent to sealing. Set the Instant Pot to Pressure Cook and cook the pork at high pressure for 30 minutes.

3. Once the Instant Pot is finished, allow the steam to release naturally for 20 minutes, then release any additional steam manually by carefully moving the vent to the venting position until the valve has dropped.

4. Preheat the oven to broil. Remove the carnitas and transfer them to a large rimmed baking sheet, then use two forks to shred the meat. Drizzle the carnitas with the oil. Broil the carnitas for 5 minutes, or until they are crispy.

5. Layer the carnitas over a bed of 1 cup (113 g) of cauliflower rice and ½ cup (38 g) of lettuce. Garnish the burrito bowls with the salsa (if using), guacamole (if using), cilantro (if using) and lime juice (if using).

(continued)

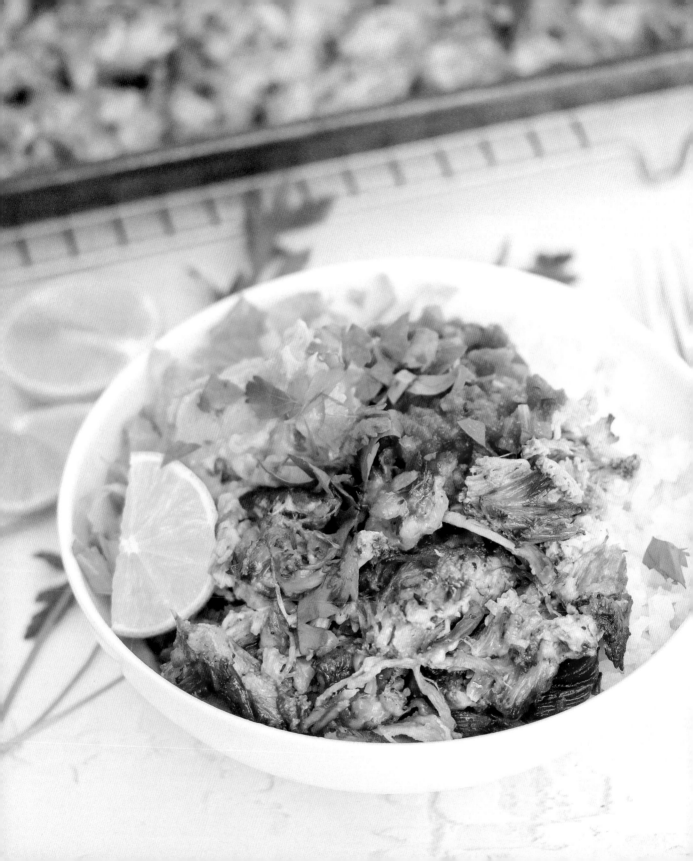

CRISPY CARNITAS BURRITO BOWLS (CONT.)

SLOW COOKER

1. Add the pork to the slow cooker and top it with the broth, orange juice, lime juice, cumin, salt, black pepper and oregano.

2. Cover the slow cooker with its lid and cook the pork on low for 6 to 8 hours or on high for 4 to 6 hours, or until the pork is cooked through and tender enough to shred.

3. Preheat the oven to broil. Transfer the carnitas to a large rimmed baking sheet, then use two forks to shred the meat. Drizzle the carnitas with the oil. Broil the carnitas for 5 minutes, or until they are crispy.

4. Layer the carnitas over a bed of 1 cup (113 g) of cauliflower rice and ½ cup (38 g) of lettuce. Garnish the burrito bowls with the salsa (if using), guacamole (if using), cilantro (if using) and lime juice (if using).

HONEY-GARLIC
TERIYAKI CHICKEN

This dish has all of the classic Asian flavors with none of the refined sugar or soy, and it's so simple to make. This sweet, sticky teriyaki chicken is a favorite in our house, served over cauliflower rice—or white rice if you eat grains—with a side of steamed broccoli. See the recipe note for a shortcut to a thickened sauce for when you're short on time!

YIELD: 6 SERVINGS

2 lbs (907 g) boneless, skinless chicken thighs, cut into 1" (2.5-cm) pieces

½ cup (120 ml) coconut aminos

3 tbsp (45 ml) honey

2 tbsp (30 ml) balsamic vinegar

2 tsp (6 g) minced garlic

½ tsp dried ginger

½ tsp salt

Pinch of red pepper flakes (optional)

Thinly sliced green onions, as needed (optional)

Sesame seeds, as needed (optional)

INSTANT POT

1. Place the chicken pieces in the Instant Pot. Add the coconut aminos, honey, vinegar, garlic, ginger and salt and stir to combine the ingredients.

2. Secure the lid on the Instant Pot in the locked position, and set the vent to sealing. Set the Instant Pot to Pressure Cook and cook the chicken at high pressure for 8 minutes.

3. Once the Instant Pot is finished, manually release the steam by carefully moving the vent to the venting position until the valve has dropped. Use a slotted spoon to transfer the chicken pieces to a large bowl. Set the bowl aside.

4. Set the Instant Pot to Sauté, and simmer the sauce until it has thickened to your liking. Pour the sauce over the chicken. Garnish the chicken with the red pepper flakes (if using), green onions (if using) and sesame seeds (if using).

(continued)

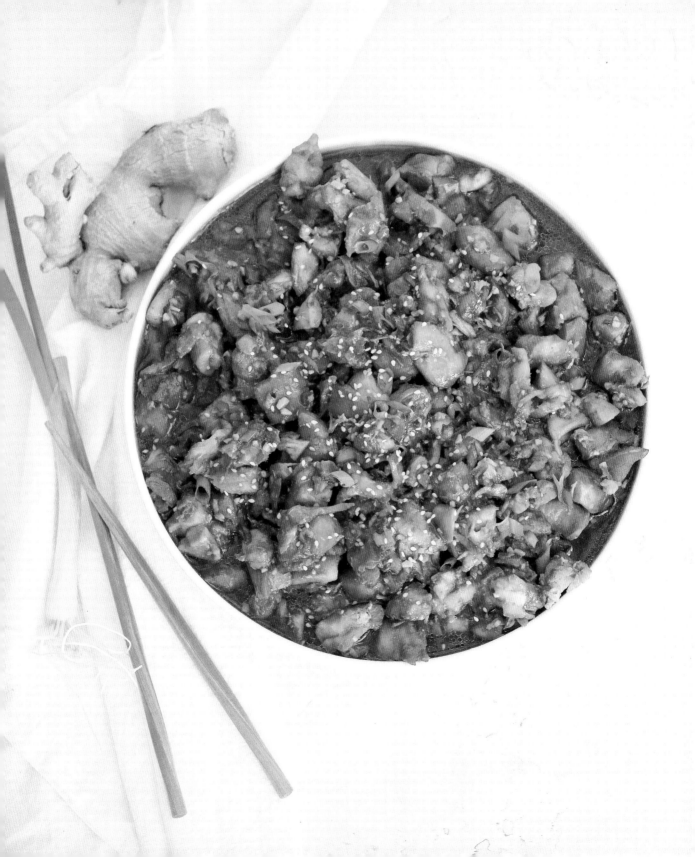

HONEY-GARLIC TERIYAKI CHICKEN (CONT.)

SLOW COOKER

1. Place the chicken pieces in the slow cooker. Add the coconut aminos, honey, vinegar, garlic, ginger and salt and stir to combine the ingredients.

2. Cover the slow cooker with its lid and cook the chicken on low for 4 hours, or until the chicken is cooked through.

3. Use a slotted spoon to transfer the chicken to a large bowl. Set the bowl aside.

4. Transfer the sauce to a medium saucepan over medium heat. Cook the sauce until it simmers, and allow it to simmer until it has thickened to your liking. Pour the sauce over the chicken. Garnish the chicken with the red pepper flakes (if using), green onions (if using) and sesame seeds (if using).

NOTE: If you're short on time and ready to serve the chicken without taking the time to reduce your sauce, try a thickener. Combine 1 tablespoon (8 g) of arrowroot flour and 1 tablespoon (15 ml) of water in a small bowl, stirring until the slurry is smooth. Stir the slurry into the sauce over low heat—it will thicken quickly.

KOREAN BARBECUE
BEEF SHORT RIBS

In this recipe, short ribs are cooked to tender, fall-off-the-bone perfection in a rich, savory Korean-style barbecue sauce. They're a little sweet, a lot savory and oh, so delicious. Flavorful food can still be simple and easy!

YIELD: 6 SERVINGS

4 lbs (1.8 kg) bone-in beef short ribs

1 tsp salt

¼ tsp black pepper

½ cup (120 ml) coconut aminos

2 tbsp (24 g) coconut sugar

1 tbsp (15 ml) rice vinegar

1 tbsp (15 ml) toasted sesame oil

1 to 2 tsp (5 to 10 ml) hot sauce

1 medium Asian pear or red apple, peeled, cored and roughly chopped

1 tbsp (9 g) minced garlic

3 green onions, thinly sliced, plus more as needed

1 (2" [5-cm]) piece fresh ginger, peeled

Cooked cauliflower rice, as needed

Toasted sesame seeds, as needed

INSTANT POT

1 Pat the short ribs dry with a paper towel and season all of the sides with the salt and black pepper. Transfer the ribs to the Instant Pot.

2 In a blender, combine the coconut aminos, sugar, vinegar, oil, hot sauce, pear, garlic, green onions and ginger. Blend until the mixture is smooth, and pour the sauce over the ribs in the Instant Pot. Stir the ribs and sauce so that the ribs are coated and the remaining sauce settles to the bottom of the pot.

3 Secure the lid on the Instant Pot in the locked position, and set the vent to sealing. Set the Instant Pot to Pressure Cook the ribs at high pressure for 45 minutes.

4 Once the Instant Pot is finished, let the pressure release naturally for 30 minutes. If any steam remains, manually release it by carefully moving the vent to the venting position until the valve has dropped. Remove the lid and transfer the ribs to a large plate.

5 Serve the ribs hot over the cauliflower rice and topped with the sauce, additional green onions and sesame seeds.

(continued)

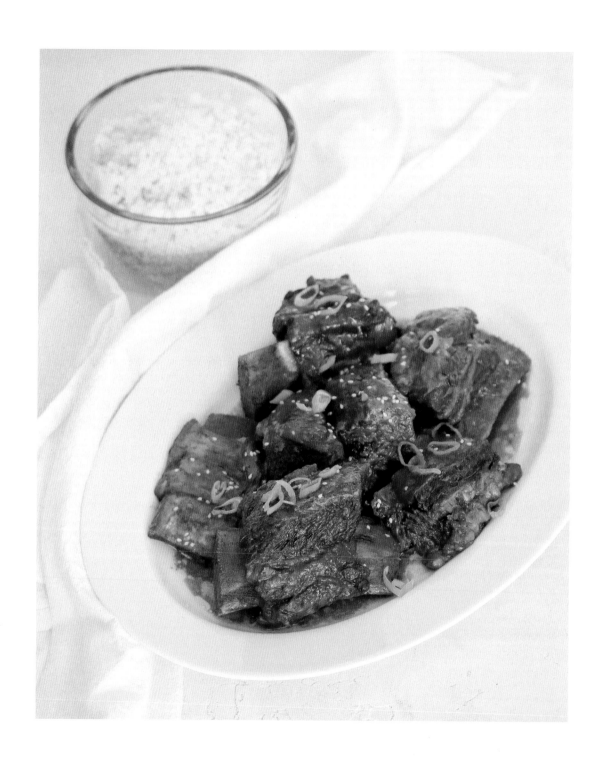

KOREAN BARBECUE BEEF SHORT RIBS (CONT.)

SLOW COOKER

1. Pat the short ribs dry with a paper towel and season all of the sides with the salt and black pepper.

2. Heat a large skillet over medium-high heat. Add the short ribs, cooking them in batches until they are browned on all sides—don't worry about cooking them completely, as we're just looking for color. Transfer the ribs to the slow cooker.

3. In a blender, combine the coconut aminos, sugar, vinegar, oil, hot sauce, pear, garlic, green onions and ginger. Blend until the mixture is smooth, and pour the sauce over the ribs in the slow cooker. Stir the ribs and sauce so that the ribs are coated and the remaining sauce settles to the bottom of the slow cooker.

4. Cover the slow cooker with its lid. Cook the ribs on low for 7 to 8 hours, or until the ribs are tender. Transfer the ribs to a large plate.

5. Serve the ribs hot over the cauliflower rice and topped with the sauce, additional green onions and sesame seeds.

LEMON CHICKEN AND RICE SOUP

Chicken soup is such a comforting, healing food—but when you add cauliflower rice and some fresh lemon, it reaches another level. This soup is fresh, warm and begging to be served with some One-Bowl Buttery Biscuits (page 115)! Try this on a chilly day, or anytime you need a light meal that will still leave you feeling nourished.

YIELD: 6 SERVINGS

1½ lbs (680 g) boneless, skinless chicken breasts or thighs

3 medium carrots, thinly sliced

3 medium ribs celery, diced

1 medium onion, finely chopped

Zest of 2 medium lemons

Juice of 2 medium lemons, plus more as needed

3 cloves garlic, minced

1½ tsp (1 g) dried parsley

1 tsp dried thyme

½ tsp dried oregano

5 cups (1.2 L) chicken broth

2 cups (227 g) fresh or frozen cauliflower rice

Salt, as needed

Black pepper, as needed

Finely chopped fresh parsley, as needed

INSTANT POT

1. Place the chicken, carrots, celery, onion, lemon zest, lemon juice, garlic, dried parsley, thyme and oregano in the Instant Pot. Add the broth and stir to combine the ingredients.

2. Secure the lid on the Instant Pot in the locked position, and set the vent to sealing. Set the Instant Pot to Pressure Cook and cook the soup at high pressure for 8 minutes.

3. Once the Instant Pot is finished, manually release the steam by carefully moving the vent to the venting position until the valve has dropped. Remove the chicken from the pot to a large cutting board or shallow dish. Use two forks to shred the chicken, then return it to the pot.

4. Set the Instant Pot to Sauté, and stir in the cauliflower rice. Simmer the soup for 2 to 3 minutes, until the cauliflower is tender. Press the Cancel button to turn off the Instant Pot. Season the soup with salt and black pepper.

5. Serve the soup hot garnished with the fresh parsley and additional lemon juice.

(continued)

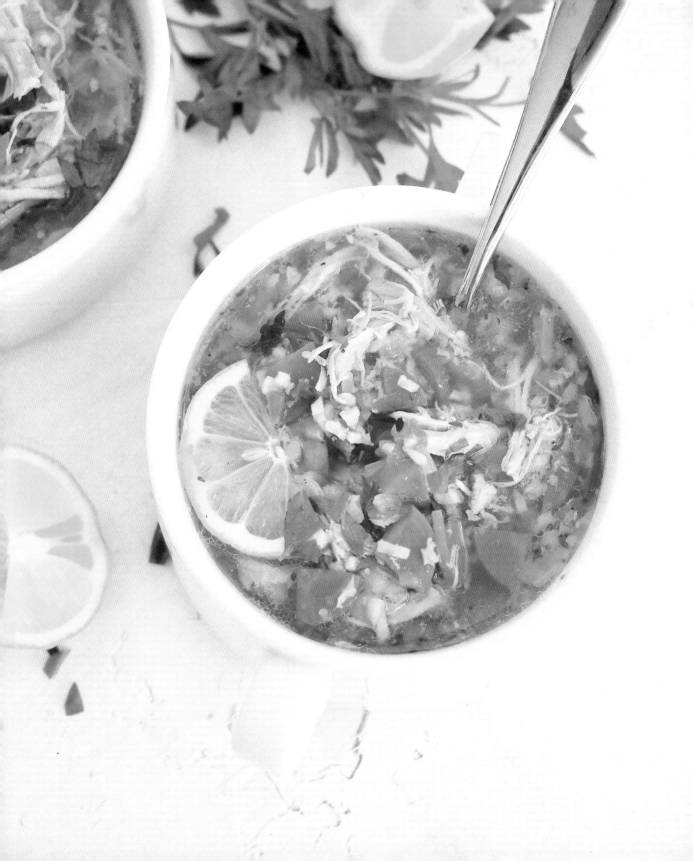

LEMON CHICKEN AND RICE SOUP (CONT.)

SLOW COOKER

1. Place the chicken, carrots, celery, onion, lemon zest, lemon juice, garlic, dried parsley, thyme and oregano in the slow cooker. Add the broth, and stir to combine the ingredients.

2. Cover the slow cooker with its lid. Cook the soup on low for 6 hours or on high for 3 to 4 hours, until the chicken is cooked through and tender enough to shred.

3. Transfer the chicken to a large cutting board or shallow dish. Use two forks to shred the chicken, then return it to the slow cooker.

4. Set the slow cooker to high and stir in the cauliflower rice. Simmer the soup for 2 to 3 minutes, until the cauliflower is tender. Turn off the heat. Season the soup with salt and black pepper.

5. Serve the soup hot garnished with the fresh parsley and additional lemon juice.

ZESTY CHICKEN FAJITA SOUP

This soup is so creamy and loaded with bold flavor that it reminds me of a stew or chowder. Smoky spices, plenty of veggies and tender shredded chicken are brought together with the secret ingredients for a rich soup: coconut milk for creaminess and nutritional yeast for a cheesy flair without the dairy. Load it up with your favorite Mexican toppings and enjoy it for days, then freeze what's left!

YIELD: 8 SERVINGS

1 tbsp (15 ml) avocado oil (for Instant Pot method)

1 medium onion, roughly chopped

1 medium green bell pepper, sliced into 1" to 2" (2.5- to 5-cm) strips

1 medium red bell pepper, sliced into 1" to 2" (2.5- to 5-cm) strips

2 tsp (6 g) minced garlic

1½ lbs (680 g) boneless, skinless chicken breasts or thighs

2 (15-oz [425-g]) cans fire-roasted diced tomatoes, with liquid

1 (4-oz [113-g]) can diced green chiles, with liquid

4 cups (960 ml) chicken broth

1 tsp onion powder

1 tsp chipotle powder

1 tsp ground cumin

1 tsp dried oregano

1 tsp smoked paprika

1 (14-oz [414-ml]) can full-fat coconut milk

¼ cup (43 g) nutritional yeast

Salt, as needed

Black pepper, as needed

Thinly sliced avocado, as needed (optional)

Roughly chopped fresh cilantro, as needed (optional)

Lime wedges, as needed (optional)

Coconut cream, as needed (optional; see Note)

INSTANT POT

1. Set the Instant Pot to Sauté, and add the oil. Once the oil is hot, add the onion, green bell pepper, red bell pepper and garlic and cook the vegetables for 2 to 3 minutes, or until they just begin to soften and brown. Press Cancel to turn off the heat. Add the chicken, tomatoes, green chiles, broth, onion powder, chipotle powder, cumin, oregano and paprika, and stir to combine the ingredients.

2. Secure the lid on the Instant Pot in the locked position, and set the vent to sealing. Set the Instant Pot to Pressure Cook and cook the mixture at high pressure for 8 minutes.

3. Once the Instant Pot is finished, allow the pressure to release naturally for 10 minutes, then manually release the remaining steam by carefully moving the vent to the venting position until the valve has dropped.

4. Transfer the chicken to a large cutting board or shallow dish. Use two forks to shred the chicken, then return it to the pot. Stir in the coconut milk and nutritional yeast. Season the soup with salt and black pepper.

5. Serve the soup hot garnished with the avocado (if using), cilantro (if using), lime wedges (if using) and a scoop of coconut cream (if using).

(continued)

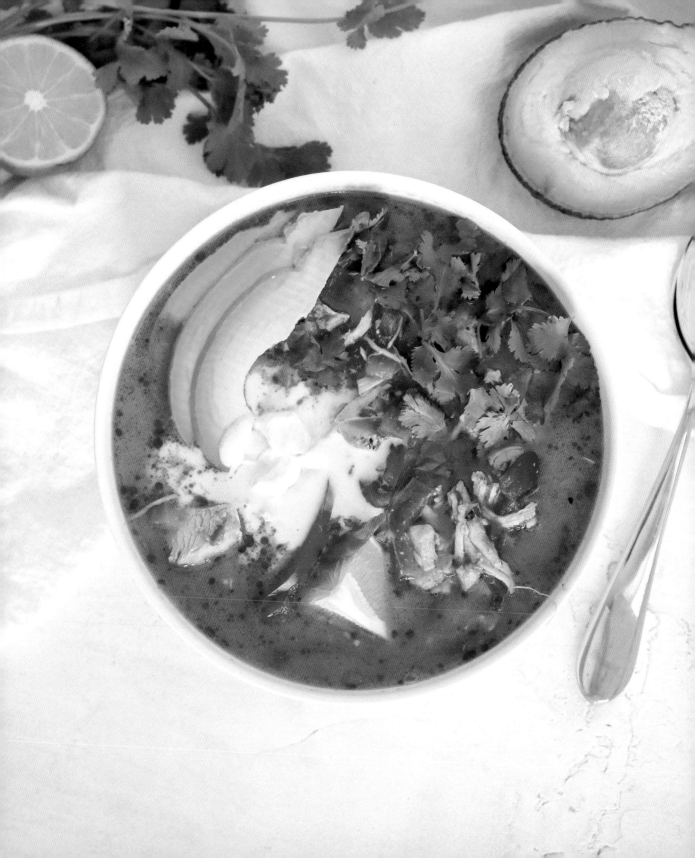

ZESTY CHICKEN FAJITA SOUP (CONT.)

SLOW COOKER

1. In the slow cooker, combine the onion, green bell pepper, red bell pepper, garlic, chicken, tomatoes, green chiles, broth, onion powder, chipotle powder, cumin, oregano and paprika, stirring the ingredients together.

2. Cover the slow cooker with its lid, and cook the mixture on low for 6 hours or on high for 3 to 4 hours, or until the chicken is cooked through and is tender enough to shred.

3. Transfer the chicken to a large cutting board or shallow dish. Use two forks to shred the chicken, then return it to the slow cooker. Stir in the coconut milk and nutritional yeast. Season the soup with salt and black pepper.

4. Serve the soup hot garnished with the avocado (if using), cilantro (if using), lime wedges (if using) and a scoop of coconut cream (if using).

NOTE: Coconut cream is the thick, rich part of the coconut milk that solidifies at the top of the can of full-fat coconut milk.

HEARTY VEGETABLE MINESTRONE

This warm, garlicky, tomato-based stew gets its bulk from tons of fresh veggies—so many, in fact, that you'll never miss the beans or grains! Serve it hot with fresh basil and a handful of Paleo-friendly crackers for an easy lunch or dinner.

YIELD: 8 SERVINGS

3 tbsp (45 ml) olive oil
(for Instant Pot method)

1 medium red bell pepper, diced

½ medium white onion, diced

8 cloves garlic, minced

3 medium ribs celery, diced

2 large carrots, thinly sliced

1 medium zucchini,
roughly chopped

1 tbsp (2 g) Italian seasoning

1 tsp salt, plus more as needed

1 tsp black pepper, plus more
as needed

2 (15-oz [425-g]) cans fire-roasted
diced tomatoes, with liquid

6 cups (1.4 L) chicken or
vegetable broth

2 cups (220 g) chopped fresh
green beans

2 cups (60 g) baby spinach,
roughly chopped

Finely chopped fresh basil,
as needed (optional)

Paleo-friendly crackers,
as needed (optional)

INSTANT POT

1. Set the Instant Pot to Sauté and add the oil. Once the oil is hot, add the bell pepper, onion, garlic, celery, carrots and zucchini. Stir and cook the vegetables for about 5 minutes, until they are slightly softened. Press Cancel to turn off the heat.

2. Add the Italian seasoning, salt, black pepper, tomatoes and broth, stirring to combine the ingredients. Stir in the green beans and spinach.

3. Secure the lid on the Instant Pot in the locked position, and set the vent to sealing. Set the Instant Pot to Pressure Cook and cook the soup at high pressure for 5 minutes.

4. Once the Instant Pot is finished, allow the pressure to release naturally for 10 minutes, then manually release the remaining steam by carefully moving the vent to the venting position until the valve has dropped. Season the soup with additional salt and black pepper.

5. Serve the soup hot garnished with the basil (if using) and with the crackers (if using) on the side.

SLOW COOKER

1. In a slow cooker, combine the bell pepper, onion, garlic, celery, carrots, zucchini, Italian seasoning, salt, black pepper, tomatoes, broth, green beans and spinach. Stir to combine the ingredients.

2. Cover the slow cooker with its lid. Cook the soup on low for 6 hours or on high for 3 to 4 hours, or until the vegetables are tender. Season the soup with additional salt and black pepper.

3. Serve the soup hot garnished with the basil (if using) and with the crackers (if using) on the side.

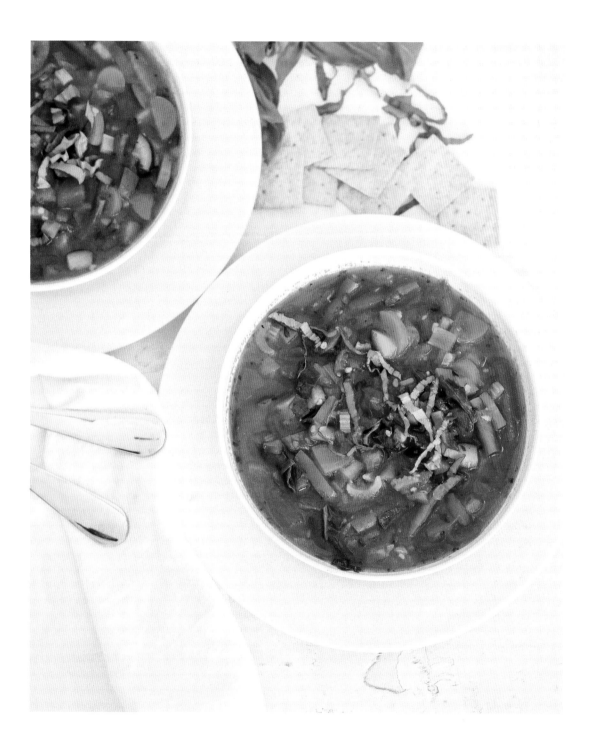

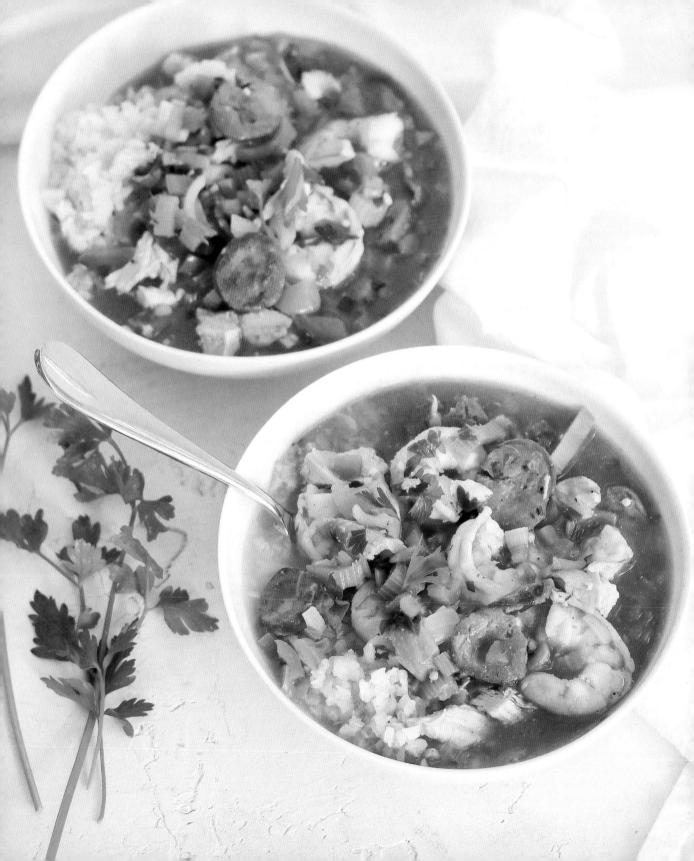

NEW ORLEANS CHICKEN, SAUSAGE AND SEAFOOD GUMBO

This dish is full of southern flair yet mild enough for the whole family to enjoy. There are plenty of veggies snuck in with the Cajun "holy trinity"—onions, green bell peppers and celery—and three types of meat for lots of texture and flavor. Enjoy it with cauliflower rice or all on its own as a hearty stew.

YIELD: 6 SERVINGS

GUMBO

¼ cup (60 ml) avocado oil

12 oz (340 g) andouille sausage, sliced into ¼" (6-mm)-thick slices

¼ cup (32 g) arrowroot flour

1 medium bunch celery (including leaves), diced

½ medium yellow onion, diced

1 medium green bell pepper, diced

4 cloves garlic, minced

6 cups (1.4 L) chicken broth

1 tsp garlic powder

1 tsp smoked paprika

½ tsp salt, plus more as needed

½ tsp black pepper, plus more as needed

½ tsp onion powder

½ tsp cayenne pepper

½ tsp dried oregano

½ tsp dried thyme

2 medium cooked boneless, skinless chicken breasts, roughly chopped

1 lb (454 g) fresh or thawed frozen shrimp, peeled and deveined

½ cup (50 g) thinly sliced green onions

½ cup (30 g) finely chopped fresh parsley

6 cups (680 g) cooked cauliflower rice

INSTANT POT

1. Set the Instant Pot to Sauté, and add the oil. Once the oil is hot, add the sausage and cook it about 2 minutes per side, until it is browned on both sides. Set the sausage aside on a plate, and add the flour to the rendered fat. Cook the mixture for 5 to 7 minutes, stirring constantly, until the arrowroot is thickened and browned. Press Cancel to turn off the heat.

2. Add the celery, onion, bell pepper and garlic and stir to combine. Stir in the broth, garlic powder, smoked paprika, salt, black pepper, onion powder, cayenne pepper, oregano and thyme.

3. Secure the lid on the Instant Pot in the locked position, and set the vent to sealing. Set the Instant Pot to Pressure Cook and cook the mixture at high pressure for 5 minutes. Once the Instant Pot is finished, manually release the steam by carefully moving the vent to the venting position until the valve has dropped.

4. Remove the lid and set the Instant Pot to Sauté. Stir in the cooked sausage, chicken and shrimp. Simmer the gumbo for about 5 minutes, until the shrimp is cooked through and looks opaque, then stir in the green onions and parsley. Season the gumbo with additional salt and black pepper.

5. Serve the gumbo hot over the cauliflower rice.

(continued)

NEW ORLEANS CHICKEN, SAUSAGE AND SEAFOOD GUMBO (CONT.)

SLOW COOKER

1. Heat the oil in a large skillet over medium-high heat. Add the sausage and cook it for about 2 minutes per side, until it is browned on both sides. Set the sausage aside on a plate, and add the flour to the rendered fat. Cook the mixture for 5 to 7 minutes, stirring constantly, until the flour is thickened and browned. Add the celery, onion, bell pepper and garlic and stir to combine the ingredients.

2. Transfer the mixture to a slow cooker. Stir in the broth, garlic powder, smoked paprika, salt, black pepper, onion powder, cayenne pepper, oregano and thyme. Cover the slow cooker with its lid and cook the mixture on low for 6 hours or on high for 3 to 4 hours, or until the vegetables are tender.

3. Remove the slow cooker's lid and, if the mixture has been cooking on low, set the temperature to high. Stir in the sausage, chicken and shrimp. Simmer the gumbo for about 5 minutes, until the shrimp is cooked through and looks opaque, then stir in the green onions and parsley. Season the gumbo with additional salt and black pepper.

4. Serve the gumbo hot over the cauliflower rice.

NOTE: To make your own at-home Cajun spice blend, combine just the garlic powder, smoked paprika, salt, black pepper, onion powder, cayenne pepper, oregano and thyme. Store the blend in an airtight container, and keep it on hand for shrimp, fish, chicken, stuffed peppers and more!

LOADED SOUTHWEST TACO SALADS

The texture and flavor of this recipe's taco meat is incredible, with a blend of rich, smoky spices and salsa for some heat and moisture—it's the best I've ever had. Double the taco meat recipe and keep it on hand for tacos, breakfast scrambles, burrito bowls and more. Making your salads ahead of time? Layer the taco meat on the bottom and the salad mix on top, and keep your dressing on the side until you're ready to serve.

YIELD: 4 SERVINGS

TACO MEAT

1 tbsp (15 ml) avocado oil

1 lb (454 g) ground beef

2 tbsp (28 g) tomato paste

1 tbsp (11 g) nutritional yeast

1 tbsp (9 g) chili powder

1½ tsp (5 g) ground cumin

1 tsp garlic powder

1 tsp onion powder

½ tsp salt

½ tsp black pepper

½ tsp dried oregano

1 cup (240 ml) salsa

INSTANT POT

1. To make the taco meat, set the Instant Pot to Sauté, and add the oil. Once the oil is hot, add the beef and cook it for 2 to 3 minutes, until it is crumbly and browned. Add the tomato paste, nutritional yeast, chili powder, cumin, garlic powder, onion powder, salt, black pepper, oregano and salsa. Stir to combine the ingredients.

2. Secure the lid on the Instant Pot in the locked position, and set the vent to sealing. Set the Instant Pot to Pressure Cook and cook the mixture at high pressure for 15 minutes.

3. Once the Instant Pot is finished, manually release the steam by carefully moving the vent to the venting position until the valve has dropped. Serve the taco meat over the taco salad (see the directions for the taco salads on the next page).

SLOW COOKER

1. To make the taco meat, heat the oil in a large skillet over medium-high heat. Add the beef and cook it for 7 to 8 minutes, until it is crumbly and browned.

2. Transfer the beef to a slow cooker. Add the tomato paste, nutritional yeast, chili powder, cumin, garlic powder, onion powder, salt, black pepper, oregano and salsa. Stir to combine the ingredients.

3. Cover the slow cooker with its lid and cook the taco meat on low for 7 to 8 hours or on high for 3 to 4 hours. Serve the taco meat over the taco salad (see the following directions for the taco salads).

(continued)

LOADED SOUTHWEST TACO SALADS (CONT.)

TACO SALADS

1 cup (240 ml) Quick Homemade Ranch (page 123) or store-bought Paleo ranch dressing

¼ cup (60 ml) hot sauce

8 cups (600 g) roughly chopped romaine lettuce

1 to 2 medium avocados, diced

½ medium red onion, finely chopped

½ cup (50 g) green onions, thinly sliced

1 medium red bell pepper, thinly sliced

Lime wedges, as needed

TACO SALADS

1. In a small bowl, whisk together the Quick Homemade Ranch and hot sauce until the dressing is smooth.

2. Divide the lettuce, avocados, red onion, green onions, bell pepper and lime wedges among four bowls or plates. Top the salads with the taco meat and dress everything with a drizzle of the spicy ranch dressing.

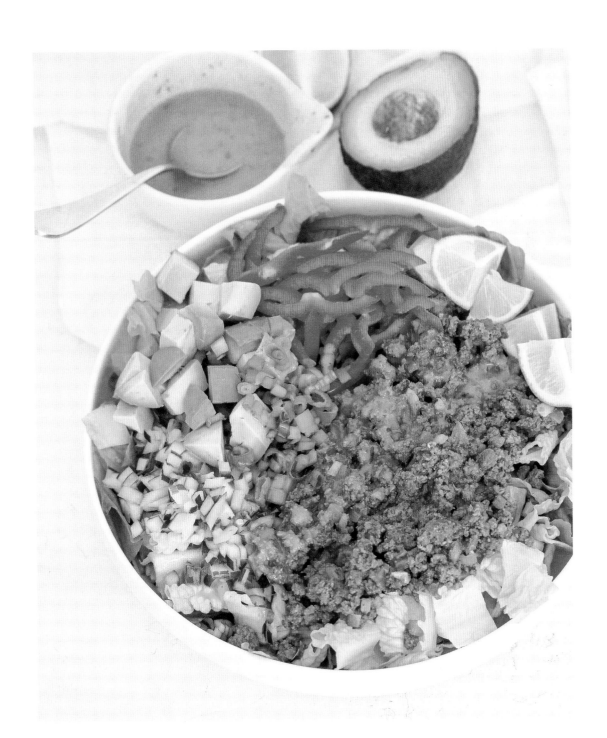

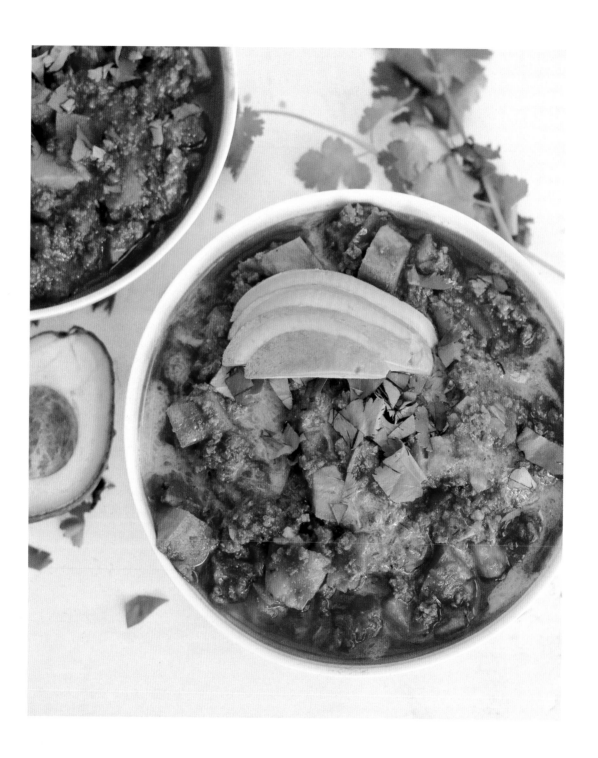

SMOKY BEEF AND SWEET POTATO CHILI

This is a family favorite: a hearty, nutrient-dense chili with mild heat and a smoky sweet barbecue flavor that will please even the pickiest of eaters. It comes together quick with just a few minutes of hands-on time and tastes even better the next day once the flavors have had the chance to marry together. I make this weekly, and I always make a double batch for plenty of leftovers!

YIELD: 6 SERVINGS

1 tbsp (15 ml) avocado oil

1 lb (454 g) ground beef

¼ medium sweet onion, diced

2 small sweet potatoes, cut into ½" (13-mm) cubes

1 (15-oz [425-g]) fire-roasted diced tomatoes, with liquid

1 (8-oz [240-ml]) can tomato sauce

¼ cup (60 ml) coconut aminos

2 tbsp (18 g) chili powder

1 tsp smoked paprika

1 tsp ground cumin

1 tsp ground cinnamon

1 tsp dried oregano

½ tsp salt

½ tsp black pepper

Quick Homemade Ranch (page 123) or store-bought Paleo ranch dressing, as needed (optional)

Diced avocado, as needed (optional)

Roughly chopped fresh cilantro, as needed (optional)

Hot sauce, as needed (optional)

INSTANT POT

1. Set the Instant Pot to Sauté, and add the oil. Once the oil is hot, add the beef. Cook the beef for 7 to 8 minutes, stirring occasionally, until it is crumbly and browned. Add the onion and sweet potatoes and stir, then press Cancel to turn off the heat. Stir in the tomatoes, tomato sauce, coconut aminos, chili powder, smoked paprika, cumin, cinnamon, oregano, salt and black pepper.

2. Secure the lid on the Instant Pot in the locked position, and set the vent to sealing. Set the Instant Pot to Pressure Cook and cook the mixture at high pressure for 14 minutes. Once the Instant Pot is finished, manually release the steam by carefully moving the vent to the venting position until the valve has dropped.

3. Serve the chili topped with the Quick Homemade Ranch (if using), avocado (if using), cilantro (if using) and hot sauce (if using).

SLOW COOKER

1. Heat the oil in a large skillet over medium-high heat. Add the beef and cook it for 7 to 8 minutes, until it is crumbly and browned. Transfer the beef to a slow cooker, and add the onion, sweet potatoes, tomatoes, tomato sauce, coconut aminos, chili powder, smoked paprika, cumin, cinnamon, oregano, salt and black pepper. Stir to combine the ingredients.

2. Cover the slow cooker with its lid and cook the chili on low for 7 to 8 hours or on high for 3 to 4 hours, or until the sweet potatoes are tender.

3. Serve the chili topped with the Quick Homemade Ranch (if using), avocado (if using), cilantro (if using) and hot sauce (if using).

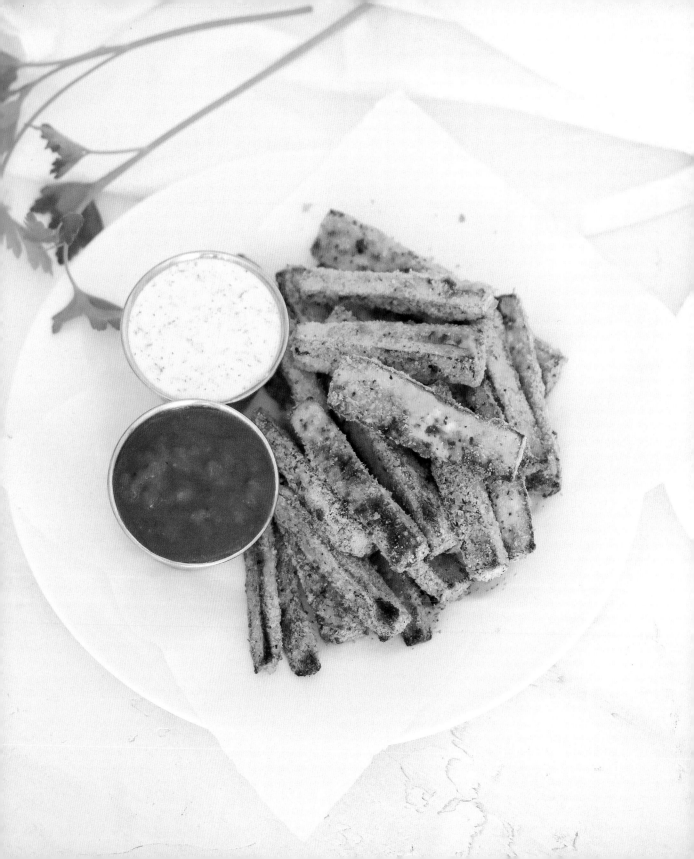

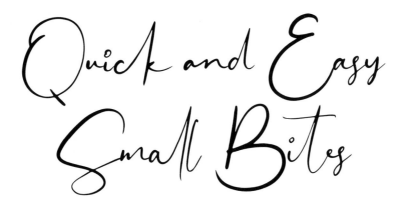

Quick and Easy Small Bites

In this chapter, you'll find some of my favorite appetizers, side dishes and "mini meals" that I come back to again and again. These are recipes that are easy to make, yet they look and taste like much more effort went into them!

Whip up a quick appetizer to impress your friends and family. Or try a savory side to complement your simplest grilled meat and veggie Paleo dishes.

I also love keeping mini meals with plenty of protein and healthy fats on hand, as they are great for snacking or when someone needs a quick lunch. Here, you'll find a few that I could eat every day!

MEDITERRANEAN CHARRED CAULIFLOWER

I was first introduced to this dish at a local restaurant, where it was served as an appetizer. One bite and I fell in love with the addicting combination of Mediterranean flavors: sweet dates, charred cauliflower, roasted pistachios, fresh dill, spicy harissa and creamy tahini. Try it as a side dish with any grilled protein, or serve it up on its own for a fun appetizer or quick lunch option.

YIELD: 6 SERVINGS

2 medium heads cauliflower, cut into bite-size florets

2 tbsp (30 ml) olive oil

½ tsp salt

¼ cup (60 ml) coconut milk

Juice of 1 medium lemon

2 to 3 tbsp (28 to 42 g) harissa

⅓ cup (75 g) tahini

3 dates, pitted and finely chopped

⅓ cup (41 g) roasted pistachios

2 tbsp (8 g) finely chopped fresh dill

1. Preheat the oven to 400°F (204°C). Place the cauliflower florets on a large rimmed baking sheet (see Note). Drizzle the oil over the cauliflower and toss them to lightly coat them with the oil. Spread the cauliflower out in a single layer and season with the salt.

2. Bake the cauliflower for 20 to 30 minutes, flipping the cauliflower halfway through the cooking time, or until the cauliflower is tender and charred.

3. In a medium bowl, whisk together the coconut milk, lemon juice, harissa and tahini.

4. Allow the cauliflower to cool for about 5 minutes, then transfer it to a large bowl. Add the dressing and toss the cauliflower to coat it with the dressing. Stir in the dates, pistachios and dill.

5. Serve the cauliflower immediately, or store leftovers in the refrigerator and serve them chilled.

NOTE: If the cauliflower will not fit on the baking sheet in a single layer, use two large rimmed baking sheets.

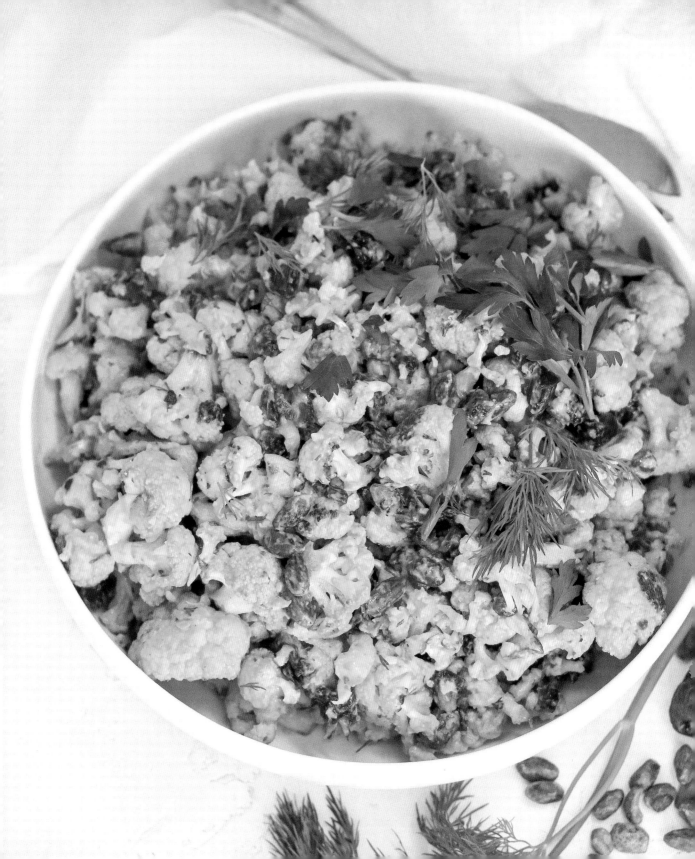

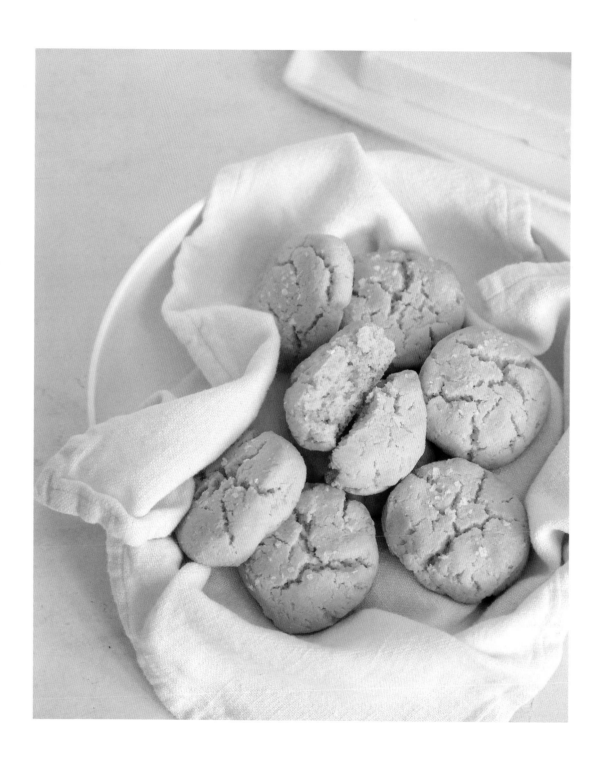

ONE-BOWL BUTTERY BISCUITS

When in doubt, make buttery biscuits! These are the perfect side dish for just about any soup, chili or holiday dish, and they are even delicious for breakfast. Biscuits and Paleo gravy, nut butter and jelly, breakfast sandwiches—you name it. Leave out the honey to take them the savory route, or leave it in for a subtly sweet flavor you'll love.

YIELD: 8 BISCUITS

2 cups (192 g) almond flour

2 large eggs

⅓ cup (80 g) grass-fed butter or ghee, melted and slightly cooled

1 tbsp (15 ml) honey (optional)

2 tsp (7 g) baking powder

½ tsp salt

Flaky sea salt, as needed (optional)

1. Preheat the oven to 350°F (177°C). Line a large baking sheet with parchment paper.

2. In a large bowl, stir together the flour, eggs, butter, honey (if using), baking powder and salt until the ingredients are just combined.

3. Use a ¼-cup (60-g) measuring cup to scoop the dough onto the prepared baking sheet. Use your hands to shape the biscuits, flattening the tops slightly. Sprinkle the tops with the flaky sea salt (if using).

4. Bake the biscuits for 18 to 20 minutes, or until they are golden.

5. Serve the biscuits warm. Store leftovers at room temperature for 2 days, covered loosely with a paper towel, or in the refrigerator for up to 1 week.

CHICKEN-APPLE-WALNUT SALAD

When you're in need of an easy make-ahead lunch or snack option, I've got you covered with this sweet and savory play on chicken salad. Nutty flavor from the walnuts, sweetness from the apples and savoriness from the chicken, celery and red onion. This chicken salad is lightly dressed in a creamy herbed ranch dressing and is ready to serve chilled anytime!

YIELD: 4 SERVINGS

3 cups (420 g) cooked and finely chopped boneless, skinless chicken breast

3 medium ribs celery, thinly sliced

1 large Granny Smith or Pink Lady apple, thinly sliced then roughly chopped

⅔ cup (77 g) roughly chopped walnuts

½ cup (120 ml) Quick Homemade Ranch (page 123) or store-bought Paleo ranch dressing

¼ cup (38 g) diced red onion

2 tbsp (8 g) finely chopped fresh parsley

½ tsp garlic powder

Salt, as needed

Black pepper, as needed

1. In a large bowl, combine the chicken, celery, apple, walnuts, Quick Homemade Ranch, onion, parsley, garlic powder, salt and black pepper. Stir until the ingredients are well combined.

2. Transfer the chicken salad to the refrigerator and chill it for 30 minutes prior to serving.

3. Serve the chicken salad chilled on its own or scooped over greens or into a lettuce wrap.

NOTE: To make this recipe extra quick, use the meat from a rotisserie chicken.

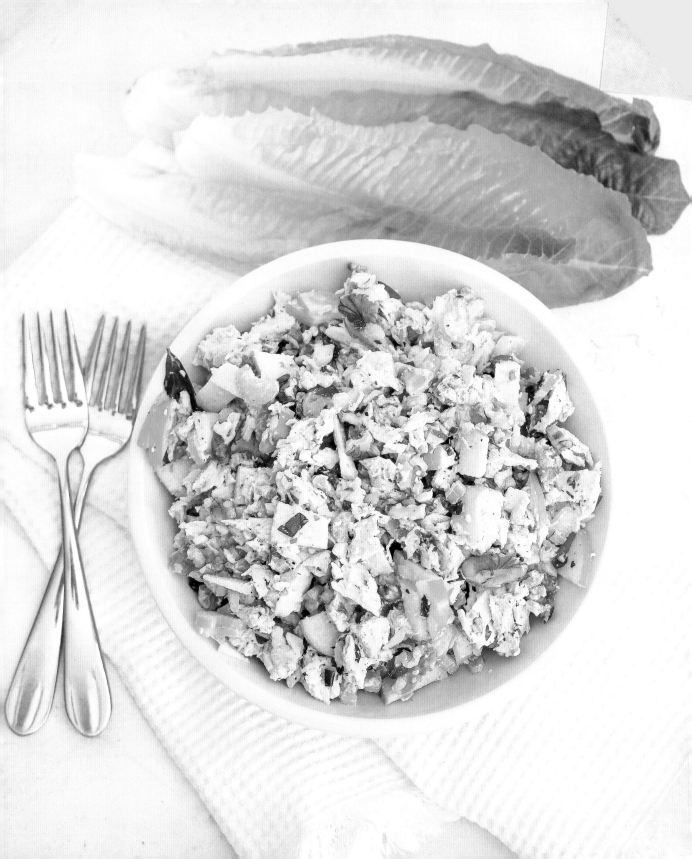

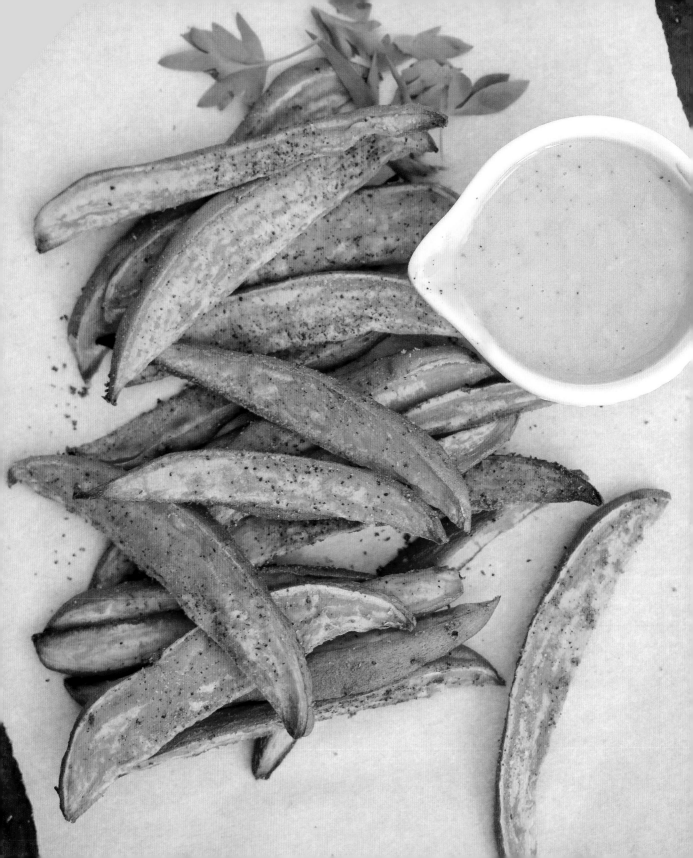

SWEET POTATO WEDGES WITH HONEY MUSTARD DIPPING SAUCE

Seasoned fries are the key to my heart, and this seasoning blend is my favorite. These fries are savory, salty, garlicky—everything good wedge fries should be. Crisp the sweet potatoes in the oven while you make a quick and creamy honey mustard dipping sauce, and the ultimate wedges are ready to go!

YIELD: 4 SERVINGS

SWEET POTATO FRIES

3 medium sweet potatoes, cut into ¼" (6-mm)-thick wedges

2 tbsp (30 ml) avocado oil or avocado oil spray

½ tsp onion powder

½ tsp garlic powder

½ tsp salt

½ tsp black pepper

HONEY MUSTARD DIPPING SAUCE

2 tbsp (23 g) cashew butter

2 tbsp (30 ml) honey or pure maple syrup

1 tbsp (16 g) Dijon mustard

¼ tsp salt

¼ tsp black pepper

1 tbsp (15 ml) unsweetened coconut or almond milk

1. To make the sweet potato fries, preheat the oven to 400°F (204°C). Line a large baking sheet with parchment paper (see Note). On the prepared baking sheet, toss the sweet potatoes with the oil, onion powder, garlic powder, salt and black pepper until the sweet potatoes are evenly coated. Arrange the sweet potatoes in a single layer on the baking sheet.

2. Bake the sweet potatoes for 30 minutes, flipping them halfway through the cooking time, or until they are lightly browned and tender.

3. To make the honey mustard dipping sauce, combine the cashew butter, honey, mustard, salt and black pepper in a small bowl, whisking until the sauce is smooth. Add the coconut milk a little at a time until the sauce reaches your preferred consistency.

4. Serve the sweet potato wedges hot with the dipping sauce.

NOTE: If the fries will not fit on the baking sheet in a single layer, use two large baking sheets.

CRISPY BAKED ZUCCHINI FRIES

When you need to use up lots of zucchini, look no further. These zucchini fries are "breaded" in a mix of almond flour and nutritional yeast for the perfect crispy coating that's completely grain- and dairy-free. They bake in the oven instead of making a mess on your stovetop, and they could not be more delicious dipped in marinara or ranch!

YIELD: 4 SERVINGS

4 medium zucchini

2 large eggs

⅔ cup (64 g) almond flour

⅓ cup (57 g) nutritional yeast

1 tsp garlic powder

1 tsp black pepper

Salt, as needed

Marinara sauce, as needed (optional)

Quick Homemade Ranch (page 123), as needed (optional)

1. Preheat the oven to 425°F (218°C). Line two large rimmed baking sheets with parchment paper and set them next to where you will be setting up your "breading" station.

2. Trim the ends off the zucchini, then slice each zucchini in half lengthwise. Slice each zucchini half into 8 pieces, for a total of 16 fries per zucchini. Place two medium shallow bowls next to the prepared baking sheets to create a breading station. In the first bowl, whisk the eggs. In the second bowl, combine the flour, nutritional yeast, garlic powder and black pepper.

3. Bread each zucchini fry by dipping it first in the eggs, then in the flour mixture, turning the fry around and tossing it lightly to coat all of its sides. Arrange the zucchini fries in a single layer on the prepared baking sheets as you go.

4. Once all zucchini fries are breaded, bake them for 20 to 25 minutes, flipping them once halfway through the cooking time, or until they are light golden brown and tender. Increase the oven temperature to broil and cook the zucchini fries for about 3 minutes, or until they are crispy, watching the fries closely so they don't burn.

5. Season the fries with salt immediately after removing them from the oven. Serve the zucchini fries hot with marinara (if using) and Quick Homemade Ranch (if using).

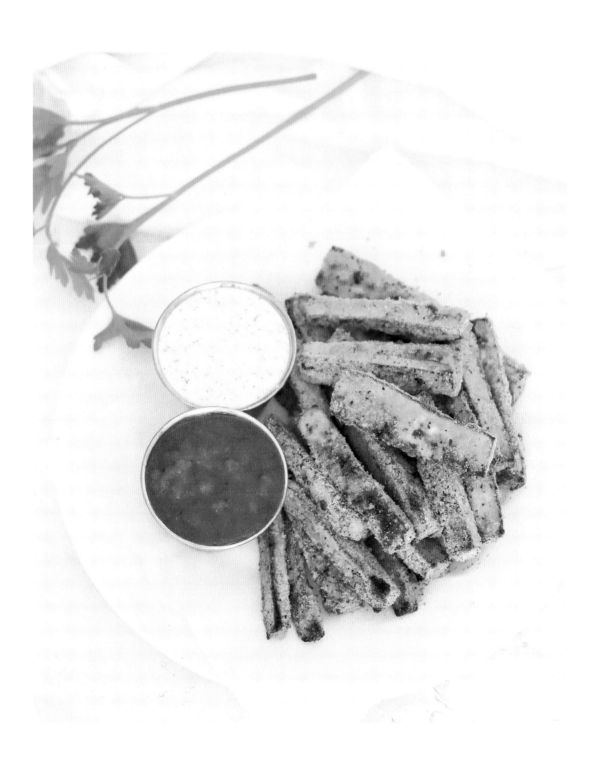

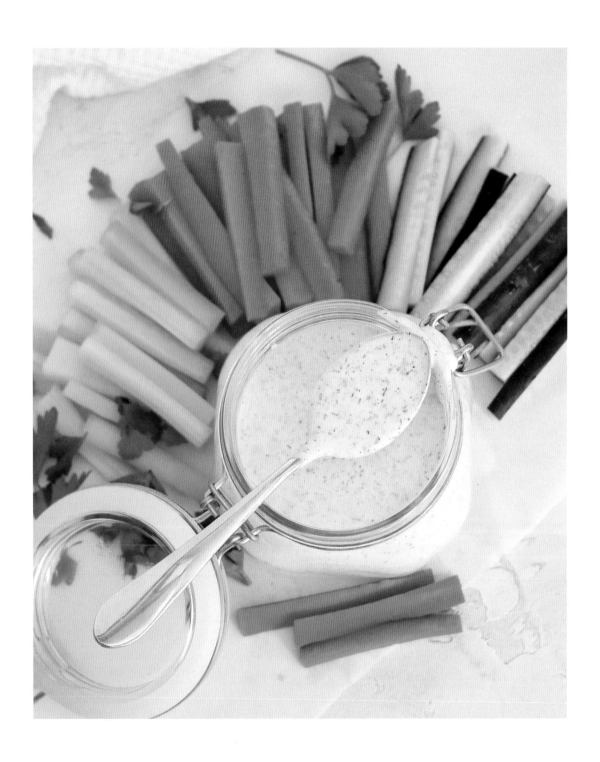

QUICK HOMEMADE RANCH

From salads to breakfast bakes, crispy chicken bites to taco skillets, you'll see I find many ways to put a good ranch dressing to use. Try this homemade version—it takes just minutes to make and tastes so much better than anything you'll buy off a shelf. I always keep a jar in the fridge. My family loves it in recipes and as a dip for fresh veggies!

YIELD: ABOUT 1 CUP (240 ML)

½ cup (110 g) Paleo mayo

¼ cup (60 ml) unsweetened coconut milk

1 tsp fresh lemon juice or apple cider vinegar

1 tsp dried parsley

1 tsp garlic powder

1 tsp onion powder

½ tsp dried dill

½ tsp dried chives

¼ tsp salt, plus more as needed

¼ tsp black pepper, plus more as needed

1. In a medium bowl, whisk together the mayo, coconut milk, lemon juice, parsley, garlic powder, onion powder, dill, chives, salt and black pepper until the dressing is smooth. Taste the dressing and season it with additional salt and black pepper. Adjust the other seasonings to taste.

2. Cover the bowl and transfer it to the refrigerator. Chill the dressing for at least 30 minutes prior to serving. Store the ranch in an airtight container in the refrigerator for up to 1 week.

CRISPY CHICKEN BITES

If the saying "you are what you eat" is true, my little brother would have surely turned into a chicken nugget at some point in our childhood. Honestly? Me too. There's just something about crispy, savory coated nuggets dipped in your favorite sauce, and I had to re-create them Paleo style so we could continue to enjoy them—guilt-free.

YIELD: 4 SERVINGS

1½ lbs (680 g) boneless, skinless chicken breasts, cut into 1" (2.5-cm) pieces

1 tsp salt, divided, plus more as needed

1 tsp black pepper, divided

1½ cups (144 g) almond flour

⅓ cup (42 g) tapioca flour

½ tsp garlic powder

3 large eggs

1 cup (240 ml) avocado oil

Quick Homemade Ranch (page 123), as needed (optional)

Honey Mustard Dipping Sauce (page 119), as needed (optional)

1. On a large cutting board, arrange the chicken pieces and season them with ½ teaspoon of the salt and ½ teaspoon of the black pepper.

2. In a large shallow bowl, combine the almond flour, tapioca flour, garlic powder and the remaining ½ teaspoon of salt and ½ teaspoon of black pepper. In a second large shallow bowl, whisk the eggs.

3. Coat the chicken pieces by dipping each piece first in the eggs, then in the flour mixture, turning it around and pressing it lightly so that it is entirely coated. Shake any excess flour off of each piece, and set the chicken aside on a plate.

4. Heat the avocado oil in a large skillet over medium heat. Add the chicken in batches, leaving a little space between each piece. Cook the chicken pieces for 2 to 3 minutes on the first side, flip them, then cook them for 1 to 2 minutes on the opposite side, or until both sides are a light golden brown and the chicken is cooked through. Place the chicken pieces on a cooling rack lined with paper towels so they stay crispy.

5. Season the chicken bites with additional salt and serve them warm with the Quick Homemade Ranch (if using) or Honey Mustard Dipping Sauce (if using).

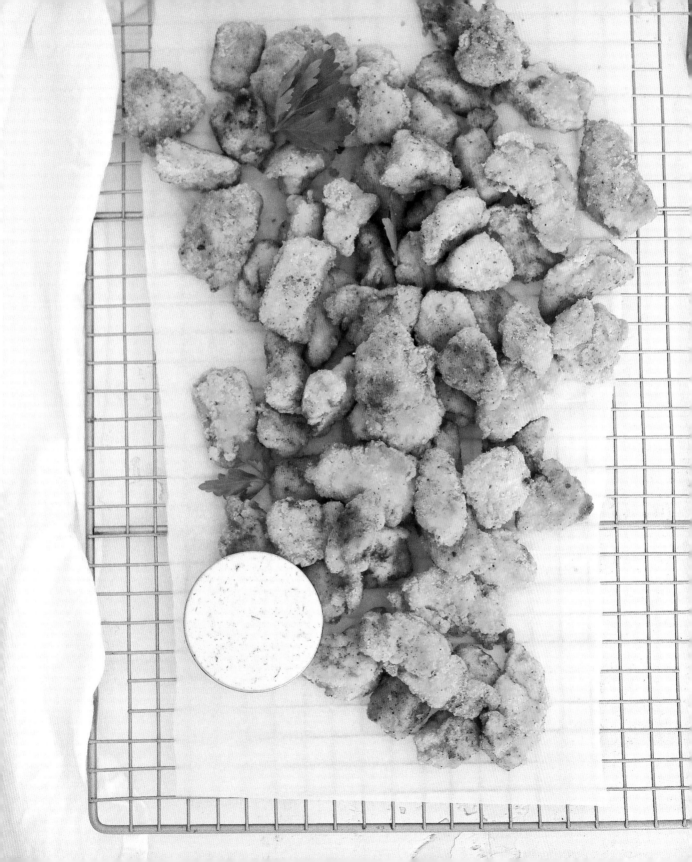

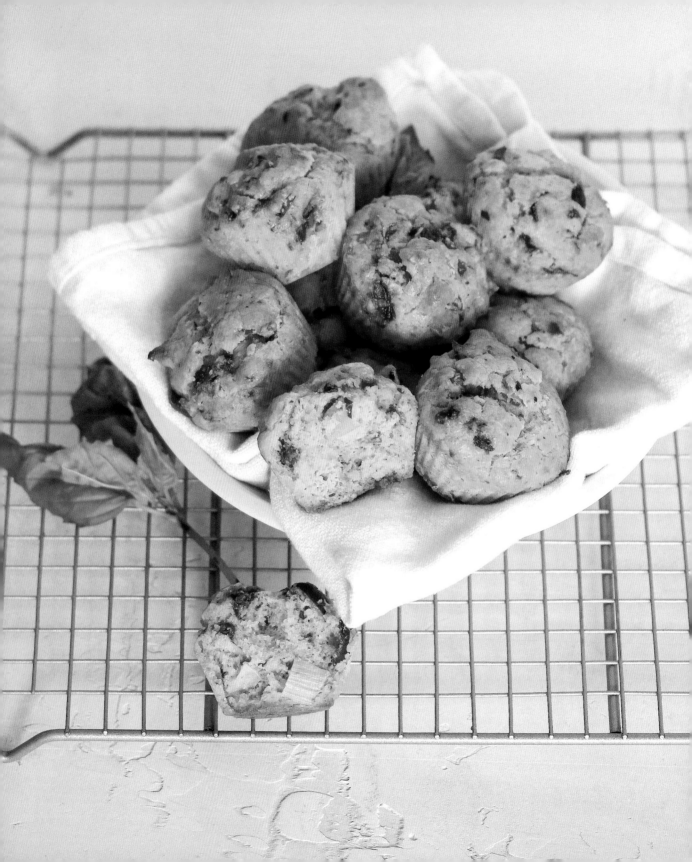

SAVORY ITALIAN PIZZA MUFFINS

Savory muffins are my favorite kind of muffins—they're warm and comforting but fill that need for something more satisfying than a sweet treat. These muffins are made Italian style, stuffed with all of the toppings you'd find on an awesome pizza, plus plenty of healthy fats. Enjoy them with pizza sauce or marinara to dip, or try them as an appetizer or quick snack or mini meal anytime.

YIELD: 12 MUFFINS

½ cup (48 g) almond flour

⅓ cup (42 g) tapioca flour

3 tbsp (24 g) coconut flour

1 tsp baking powder

½ tsp salt

½ tsp garlic powder

¼ tsp dried oregano

3 large eggs, beaten

⅓ cup (80 ml) olive oil

⅓ cup (46 g) pepperoni slices, roughly chopped

¼ cup (42 g) drained, roughly chopped marinated artichoke hearts

¼ cup (14 g) diced sun-dried tomatoes

3 tbsp (24 g) sliced black olives

Pizza or marinara sauce, as needed (optional)

1. Preheat the oven to 350°F (177°C). Line a 12-well muffin pan with parchment paper liners.

2. In a large bowl, stir together the almond flour, tapioca flour, coconut flour, baking powder, salt, garlic powder and oregano until the ingredients are mixed well. Add the eggs, oil, pepperoni, artichoke hearts, tomatoes and olives and stir until the ingredients are just combined. Use a spoon or a cookie scoop to fill each muffin well almost to the top.

3. Bake the muffins for 20 to 25 minutes, or until they are golden on top and firm in the center. Allow the muffins to cool in the muffin pan, then transfer them to a cooling rack.

4. Serve the muffins warm with the pizza sauce for dipping (if using). Store leftover muffins at room temperature for 2 days, covered loosely with a paper towel, or for up to 1 week in an airtight container in the refrigerator.

HAWAIIAN SALMON AND AVOCADO POKE

Poke is a favorite around my house for its light, flavorful sauce and fresh ingredients. Tuna is great, but salmon always takes the cake in my book. I grew up eating tons of salmon, and I love it in a good poke. Try this recipe as an appetizer with plantain chips, or serve it on its own for an easy, light meal.

YIELD: 4 SERVINGS

1 lb (454 g) sushi-grade salmon, cut into ½" (13-mm) cubes

2 tbsp (30 ml) coconut aminos

1½ tbsp (23 ml) toasted sesame oil

½ tsp salt

1 large avocado, cubed

½ cup (67 g) diced cucumber

2 green onions, thinly sliced

1½ tbsp (15 g) toasted sesame seeds

1. Place the salmon in a large bowl. Add the coconut aminos, oil and salt. Use your hands or a large spoon to gently toss the ingredients together.

2. Add the avocado, cucumber, green onions and sesame seeds and toss again to lightly coat the ingredients in the sauce.

3. Serve the poke on its own, over cauliflower rice or as a "dip" with plantain chips.

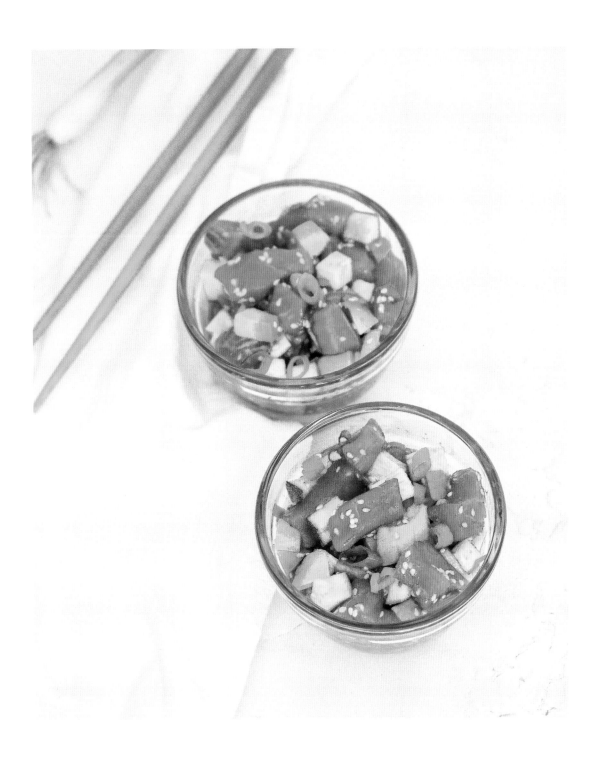

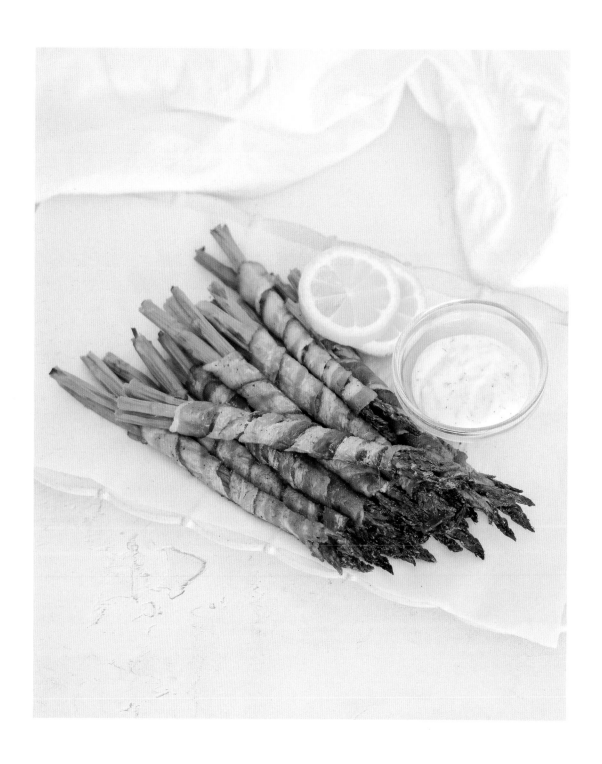

ROASTED BACON-WRAPPED ASPARAGUS

Fresh asparagus spears are wrapped in smoky bacon and roasted to perfection to make this easy appetizer that also works great as a side dish. Serve it alone or with my simple Lemon-Garlic Aioli for a flavor explosion—and try not to eat the whole plate!

YIELD: 4 SERVINGS

BACON-WRAPPED ASPARAGUS

60 thin or 40 thick asparagus spears

Avocado oil spray or avocado oil, as needed

½ tsp salt

½ tsp black pepper

10 slices of bacon

LEMON-GARLIC AIOLI

⅓ cup (73 g) Paleo mayo

Juice of ½ medium lemon

1 tsp minced garlic

1 tsp finely chopped fresh parsley

¼ tsp salt

¼ tsp black pepper

1. To make the bacon-wrapped asparagus, preheat the oven to 400°F (204°C). Line a large baking sheet with parchment paper or foil and place a wire rack on top so the bacon drains and stays crisp while baking.

2. Lightly spray the asparagus spears with the avocado oil spray. Season them with the salt and pepper, then toss them to coat them in the oil and seasonings. Slice the bacon strips lengthwise to make 20 thin slices.

3. Wrap a slice of bacon around 3 thin asparagus spears or 2 thick spears. Keep the bacon in a single, flat layer as you wrap it around the asparagus and don't allow it to overlap. Lay the wrapped asparagus bundles on the prepared baking sheet, making sure that they aren't touching and the ends of the bacon slices are on the bottom of the bundles.

4. Bake the asparagus for 25 minutes, or until the bacon is cooked and the asparagus is tender. Increase the oven temperature to broil and cook the asparagus for 2 to 3 minutes to finish crisping the bacon, watching closely so it doesn't burn.

5. To make the lemon-garlic aioli, combine the mayo, lemon juice, garlic, parsley, salt and black pepper in a small bowl, whisking until the aioli is smooth. Serve the bacon-wrapped asparagus warm with the aioli for dipping.

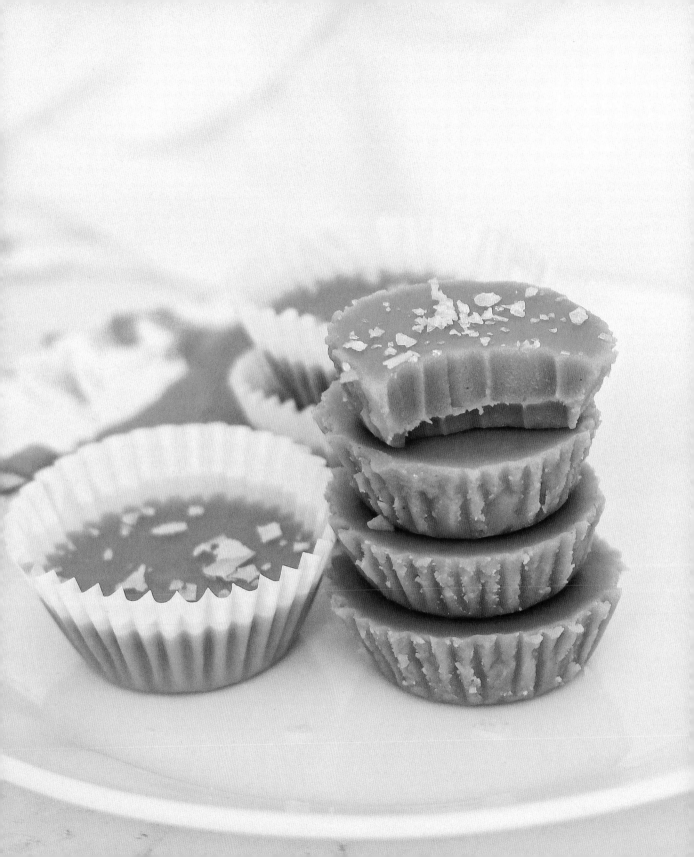

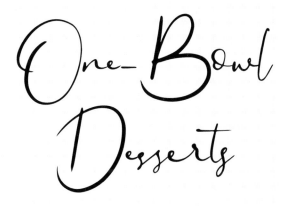

One-Bowl Desserts

Everyone loves dessert—and a Paleo-friendly one that tastes like the "real deal"? I just can't say no! This chapter is filled with my favorite one-bowl wonders that will convince any non-Paleo eater that healthy can absolutely be delicious.

While you can make each of these recipes with—that's right—just one bowl, a couple of desserts have options for an additional drizzle or glaze. Just know that even if you stick with the basic recipe, you're in for a treat!

SALTED CHOCOLATE CHUNK COOKIES

Everyone needs the perfect chocolate chip cookie in their life, and this is the Paleo version. I often make the dough ahead of time and keep it in the fridge or freezer for baking up a few of these cookies anytime my family is in the mood. They're chewy, crisp, soft in the center—and with the chunks of gooey chocolate and sea salt flakes on top, you're going to need a double batch!

YIELD: 12 COOKIES

½ cup (120 g) grass-fed butter or coconut oil, softened

¾ cup (144 g) coconut sugar

1 tsp pure vanilla extract

1 large egg

2¼ cups (216 g) almond flour

½ tsp baking soda

½ tsp salt

⅔ cup (120 g) dairy-free semisweet chocolate chunks or roughly chopped dark chocolate, plus more as needed

Flaky sea salt, as needed

1. In a large bowl, use a fork or whisk to mix together the butter, sugar and vanilla until the ingredients are smooth. Stir in the egg. Add the flour, baking soda and salt, and stir until the ingredients are just combined. Fold in the chocolate chunks. Transfer the dough to the refrigerator for 30 to 60 minutes or up to overnight to firm up.

2. Preheat the oven to 350°F (177°C). Line a large baking sheet with parchment paper.

3. Use a cookie scoop to scoop 12 balls of dough onto the prepared baking sheet. Press down on each slightly to flatten the top, and top each cookie with a few extra chocolate chunks and a sprinkle of sea salt.

4. Bake the cookies for 10 minutes, or until they are golden brown around the edges. They will continue to firm up on the baking sheet as they cool. Allow the cookies to cool for 5 minutes on the baking sheet before transferring them to a wire cooling rack to cool completely.

5. Store leftover cookies at room temperature, covered loosely with a paper towel, or in the refrigerator for up to 4 days.

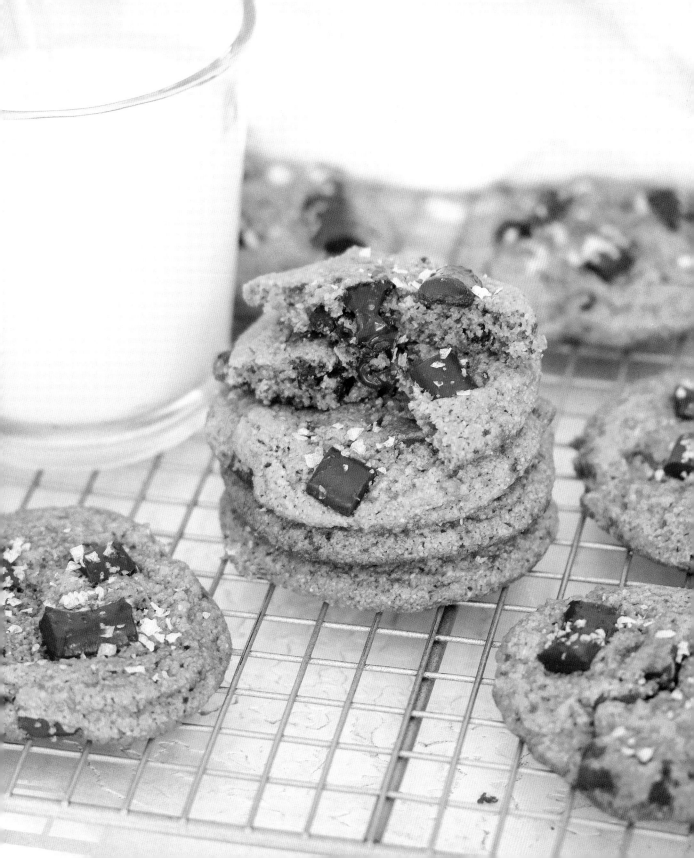

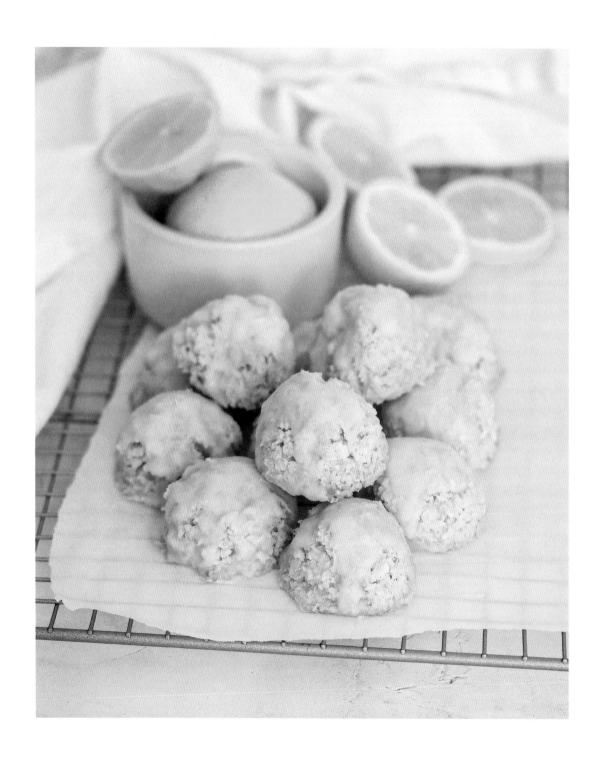

LEMON-COCONUT MACAROONS

Light, fluffy, sweet and tart: all of the things a good lemon dessert should be. These macaroons are made with simple ingredients and are so easy to make. Eat them as is for a one-bowl recipe, or grab an extra small bowl and dress them up with a tart lemon glaze for an additional boost of flavor.

YIELD: 15 MACAROONS

MACAROONS

1½ cups (114 g) unsweetened shredded coconut

½ cup (48 g) almond flour

½ cup (120 ml) pure maple syrup

¼ cup (60 g) coconut butter, melted

2 tbsp (30 ml) fresh lemon juice

Zest of 1 medium lemon

1 tsp pure vanilla extract

¼ tsp salt

GLAZE (OPTIONAL)

2 tbsp (30 g) coconut butter

1 tbsp (15 ml) pure maple syrup

2 tbsp (30 ml) fresh lemon juice

2 tbsp (30 g) coconut oil

Lemon zest, as needed

1. To make the macaroons, preheat the oven to 275°F (135°C). Line a large baking sheet with parchment paper.

2. In a large bowl, stir together the coconut, flour, maple syrup, coconut butter, lemon juice, lemon zest, vanilla and salt. Use a cookie scoop to create a macaroon shape, packing the dough into the scoop so one side is flat. Release the dough onto the baking sheet, flat side down. Repeat this process until you have 15 macaroons.

3. Bake the macaroons for 35 to 40 minutes, or until the macaroons are light golden brown on the bottom and hold together in the center.

4. While the macaroons cool, make the glaze (if using). In a small saucepan over medium-low heat, melt together the coconut butter, maple syrup, lemon juice and oil. Alternatively, combine the ingredients in a small microwave-safe bowl and warm them for 30 seconds in the microwave. Whisk the ingredients until they are smooth. Allow the glaze to cool and thicken just slightly, until it's easy to drizzle with a spoon.

5. Drizzle the glaze over the macaroons, then top them with the lemon zest for extra lemon flavor. Allow the glaze to harden, then serve. Store the macaroons in an airtight container in the refrigerator for up to 1 week.

FUDGY CHOCOLATE-WALNUT BROWNIES

You know those brownies that are soft and fudgy on the inside and have that crinkly, crackled crust on the outside that's just a little chewy, a little crisp? These are those brownies. They're absolutely perfect in every way and better than any boxed mix!

YIELD: 9 OR 16 BROWNIES

1 cup (180 g) dairy-free semisweet chocolate chips

6 tbsp (90 g) grass-fed butter or ghee

1 cup (192 g) coconut sugar

1 tsp pure vanilla extract

½ tsp salt

2 large eggs

½ cup (48 g) almond flour

¼ cup (28 g) cacao powder

½ cup (58 g) roughly chopped walnuts

1. Preheat the oven to 350°F (177°C). Line a 9-inch (23-cm) glass baking dish with parchment paper.

2. Using the microwave for 30 seconds at a time, or a double boiler on the stove, heat the chocolate chips and butter until the chocolate is just melted. Stir the mixture and add the sugar, vanilla and salt. Stir in the eggs, flour, cacao powder and walnuts until the ingredients are just combined. Don't overmix the batter.

3. Scoop the batter into the prepared baking dish and smooth the top. Bake the brownies for 30 to 35 minutes, or until the edges are crisp and the center is set.

4. Allow the brownies to cool completely before slicing them into squares. I recommend letting them come to room temperature then transferring them to the refrigerator for about 30 minutes so they firm up completely.

5. Serve the brownies at room temperature or chilled for a fudgy texture. Store leftovers in an airtight container in the refrigerator for up to 1 week.

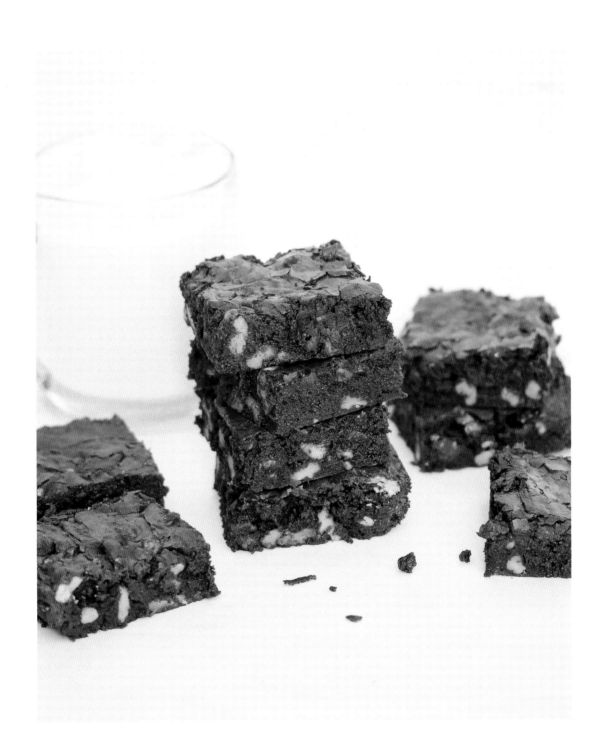

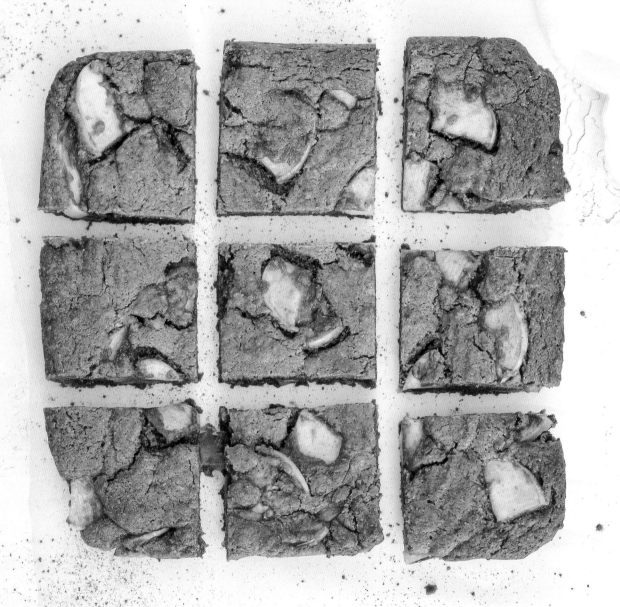

CINNAMON APPLE PIE BLONDIES

Blondies and apple pie are a match made in heaven, and they come together so perfectly in this simple dessert. If apple pie is your thing, but you're not keen on baking, this recipe is for you. Creating that apple pie flavor can be quick and easy!

YIELD: 9 BLONDIES

¾ cup (144 g) coconut sugar

½ cup (90 g) cashew or almond butter

¼ cup (60 g) grass-fed butter or coconut oil, melted

1 large egg

2 tsp (10 ml) pure vanilla extract

1 cup (96 g) almond flour

2 tsp (6 g) ground cinnamon

1 tsp baking soda

½ tsp salt

1 medium Pink Lady or Granny Smith apple, cored and thinly sliced then roughly chopped, divided

1. Preheat the oven to 350°F (177°C). Line a 9-inch (23-cm) glass baking dish with parchment paper.

2. In a medium bowl, stir together the sugar, cashew butter, melted butter, egg and vanilla until the ingredients are smooth. Stir in the flour, cinnamon, baking soda and salt. Fold in three-fourths of the apple slices.

3. Transfer the batter to the prepared baking dish and smooth the top. Top the batter with the remaining one-fourth of the apple slices. Bake the blondies for 20 to 25 minutes, or until the top is light golden brown and the center is set.

4. Allow the blondies to cool completely before slicing them into squares. I recommend letting them come to room temperature then transferring them to the refrigerator for about 30 minutes so they firm up completely.

5. Serve the blondies chilled or at room temperature. Store leftovers in an airtight container in the refrigerator for up to 1 week.

BAKED CRISP-STUFFED APPLES

These stuffed apples will leave your home smelling like heaven and your taste buds begging for more. Chopped nuts, coconut sugar and cinnamon are combined with butter or coconut oil to create the perfect "crisp" filling that gets stuffed inside of fresh apples. The apples are baked in water so they come out tender and juicy. Don't forget the dairy-free ice cream!

YIELD: 4 SERVINGS

2 large Pink Lady apples

⅓ cup (39 g) finely chopped walnuts or pecans

⅓ cup (64 g) coconut sugar

⅓ cup (32 g) almond flour

3 tbsp (14 g) unsweetened shredded coconut

3 tbsp (45 ml) melted butter or coconut oil

1 tsp ground cinnamon

½ tsp salt

Dairy-free ice cream (optional)

1. Preheat the oven to 350°F (177°C). Fill a 9-inch (23-cm) glass baking dish with 1 inch (2.5 cm) of water.

2. Slice each apple down the middle and use a cookie scoop, metal spoon or melon baller to scoop out the middle of the apple. Remove the seeds and stem, and keep scooping until there is a 3-inch (7.5-cm)-wide well in the center of each half of the apple for the filling. Be careful not to scoop too far down and puncture through the bottom side of the apple.

3. In a medium bowl, stir together the walnuts, sugar, flour, coconut, butter, cinnamon and salt.

4. Divide the filling between the four apple halves, and place the apples filling side up in the prepared baking dish.

5. Bake the apples for 45 minutes, or until the apples are tender and the filling is crisp and golden brown. Enjoy the apples hot served on their own or with a scoop of dairy-free ice cream.

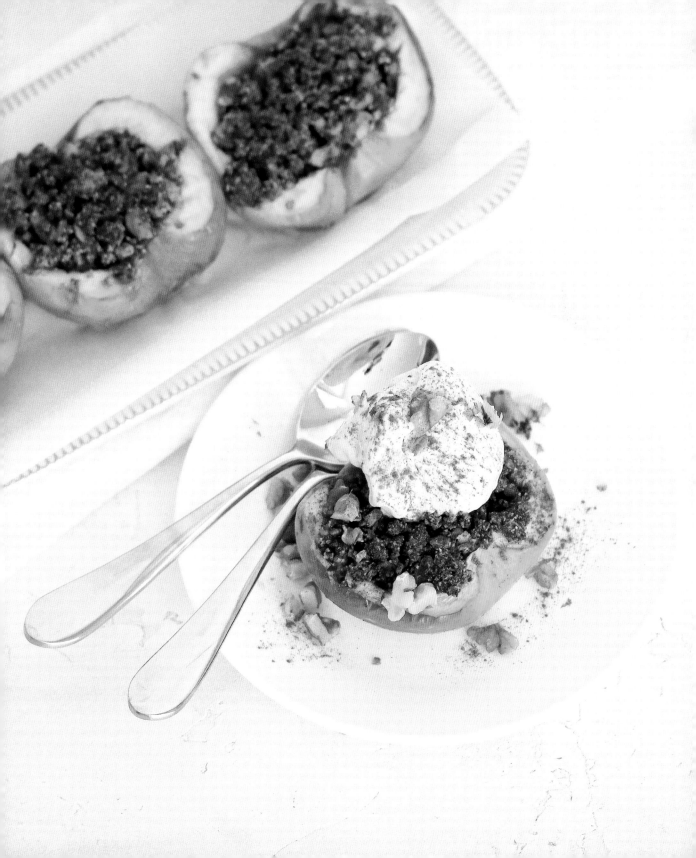

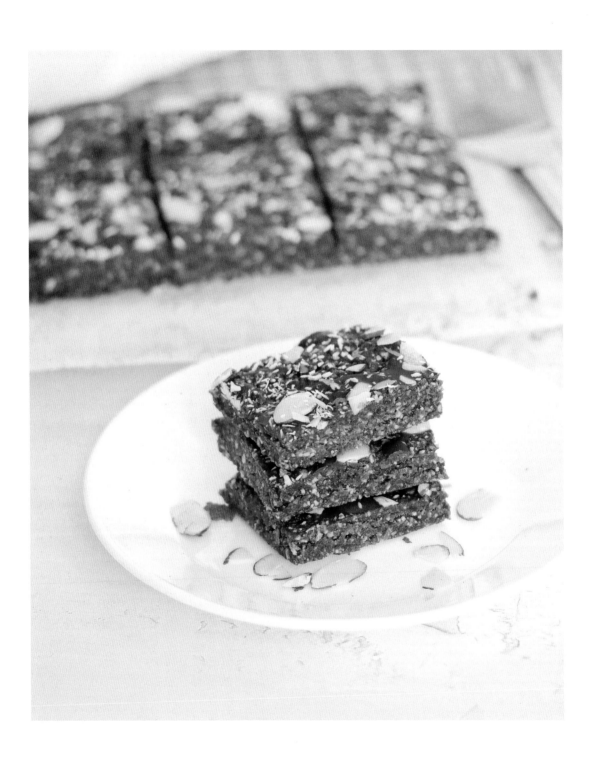

NO-BAKE GERMAN CHOCOLATE CAKE BARS

Homemade fruit and nut bars were my specialty in college—I made every flavor combination you can imagine, and I would not only pack them for myself for long days of internships and night classes but also gift them to friends and family. Food really is my love language! These bars taste just like German chocolate cake with the coconut, pecans and almond extract, which is the exact flavor I brought as a gift for my now-husband when we met up for our first "real" date! Keep these bars simple with my one-bowl method, or add an extra chocolate drizzle on top if you're feeling fancy.

YIELD: 9 TO 16 BARS

CAKE BARS

1 cup (121 g) pecans

1 cup (110 g) sliced almonds, plus more as needed

15 pitted Medjool dates

¾ cup (57 g) unsweetened shredded coconut

1 tsp pure vanilla extract

¼ tsp pure almond extract

2 tbsp (14 g) cacao powder

½ tsp salt

CHOCOLATE DRIZZLE (OPTIONAL)

¼ cup (45 g) dairy-free semisweet chocolate chips

2 tsp (10 g) coconut oil

1. To make the cake bars, line a 9-inch (23-cm) glass baking dish with parchment paper.

2. In a food processor, combine the pecans, almonds, dates, coconut, vanilla, almond extract, cacao powder and salt. Pulse until the dates are broken down and the mixture starts to resemble a dough. Scrape down the sides of the processor and pulse a few more times to fully combine the ingredients.

3. Transfer the mixture to the prepared baking dish, pressing it down into the dish and smoothing the top.

4. To make the chocolate drizzle (if using), heat the chocolate chips and oil in the microwave for 30 seconds at a time, or in a double boiler on the stove until the chocolate is just melted. Whisk to combine the ingredients. Drizzle the chocolate over the top of the bars with a small spoon, then sprinkle the bars with a few extra almonds.

5. Transfer the dish to the refrigerator and let the bars chill until they are firm. Slice the bars into 9 to 16 squares, and serve them chilled. Store leftovers in an airtight container in the refrigerator for up to 2 weeks.

CHOCOLATE CHIP "OATMEAL" COOKIE DOUGH

Somehow, the cookie dough is always better than the actual cookie. This sweet treat brings you that unbaked cookie dough in all its glory but without any eggs, so it's ready to be eaten as-is anytime. I use shredded coconut for the perfect "oatmeal" texture without the grains and load the dough with chocolate chips.

YIELD: 12 SERVINGS

¾ cup (57 g) unsweetened shredded coconut

⅓ cup (60 g) dairy-free semisweet chocolate chips

½ cup (48 g) almond flour

½ cup (90 g) cashew butter

¼ cup (48 g) coconut sugar

1 tsp pure vanilla extract

¼ tsp salt

1. In a medium bowl, stir together the coconut, chocolate chips, flour, cashew butter, sugar, vanilla and salt.

2. Roll the cookie dough into 12 balls, or store it in a bowl as is. Transfer the cookie dough to the fridge, and serve it chilled. Store the cookie dough in an airtight container in the refrigerator for up to 2 weeks.

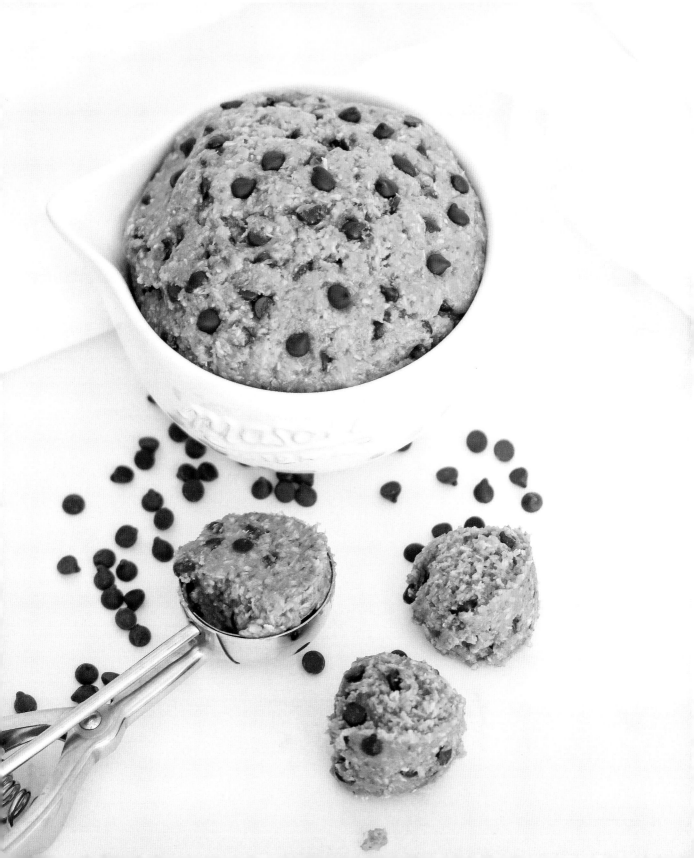

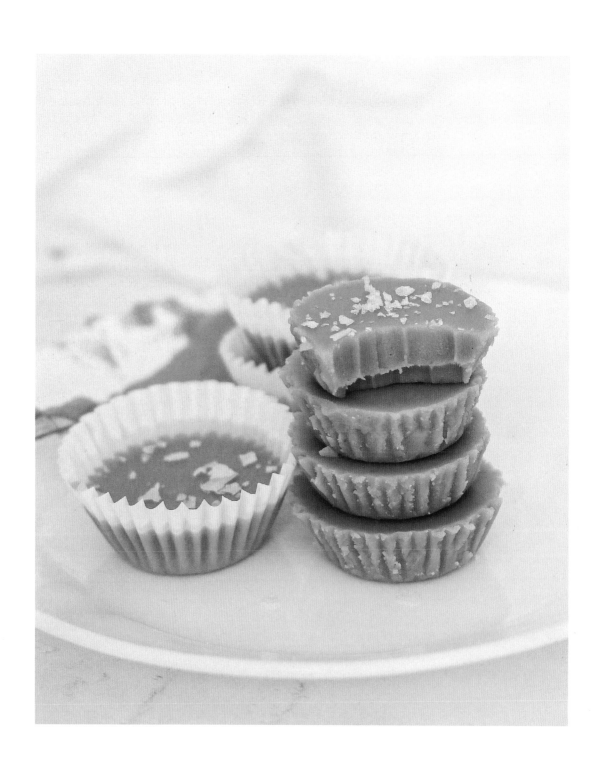

MAPLE FUDGE FAT BOMBS

Healthy fats are what make a dessert truly satisfying and not just a sugar bomb leaving you with a crash. Next time you're hit with a craving, grab one of these bites and give yourself a dose of brain fuel and a hint of sweetness at the same time. These are delicious straight out of the fridge or even blended into your coffee!

YIELD: 12 FAT BOMBS

¼ cup (45 g) cashew or almond butter

2 tbsp (30 g) grass-fed butter or ghee

1 tbsp (15 g) coconut oil

2 tsp (10 ml) pure maple syrup

Flaky sea salt, as needed

1. Line a mini muffin pan with 12 parchment paper liners.

2. Using the microwave for 30 seconds at a time, until just melted, or a double boiler on the stove, heat the cashew butter, grass-fed butter, oil and maple syrup until the ingredients are melted and smooth. Stir the ingredients together to combine.

3. Pour the mixture into the prepared mini muffin pan. Sprinkle the tops with the sea salt. Transfer the mini muffin pan to the refrigerator, and chill the fat bombs until they are firm.

4. Store the fat bombs in an airtight container in the refrigerator for up to 2 weeks.

CHOCOLATE-CHERRY ALMOND CLUSTERS

These no-bake clusters are simple to make, and I always thank my past self when I open the fridge at night and remember I have these waiting for me! They're the perfect combination of chocolatey, salty, tart and sweet, and just one cluster fixes any cravings fast.

YIELD: 20 CLUSTERS

½ cup (90 g) dairy-free semisweet or dark chocolate chips

1 tbsp (15 g) coconut oil

½ tsp pure vanilla extract

1½ cups (255 g) roasted almonds

¾ cup (120 g) dried cherries

Flaky sea salt, as needed

1. Line a large baking sheet with parchment paper.

2. Using the microwave for 30 seconds at a time or a double boiler on the stove, heat the chocolate chips and coconut oil until the chocolate is just melted. Stir in the vanilla, then allow the mixture to cool for about 2 minutes, until the chocolate thickens slightly.

3. Stir in the almonds and cherries until they are coated with the chocolate.

4. Spoon mounds of the mixture onto the prepared baking sheet and sprinkle them with the sea salt. Transfer the baking sheet to the refrigerator and chill the clusters for 30 minutes, or until the chocolate is set.

5. Store the clusters in an airtight container in the refrigerator for up to 2 weeks.

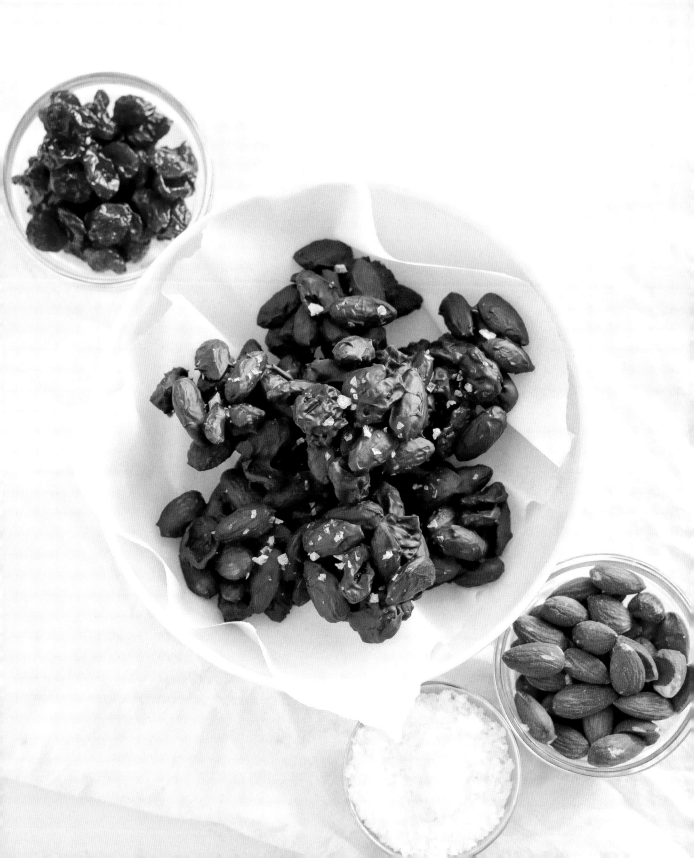

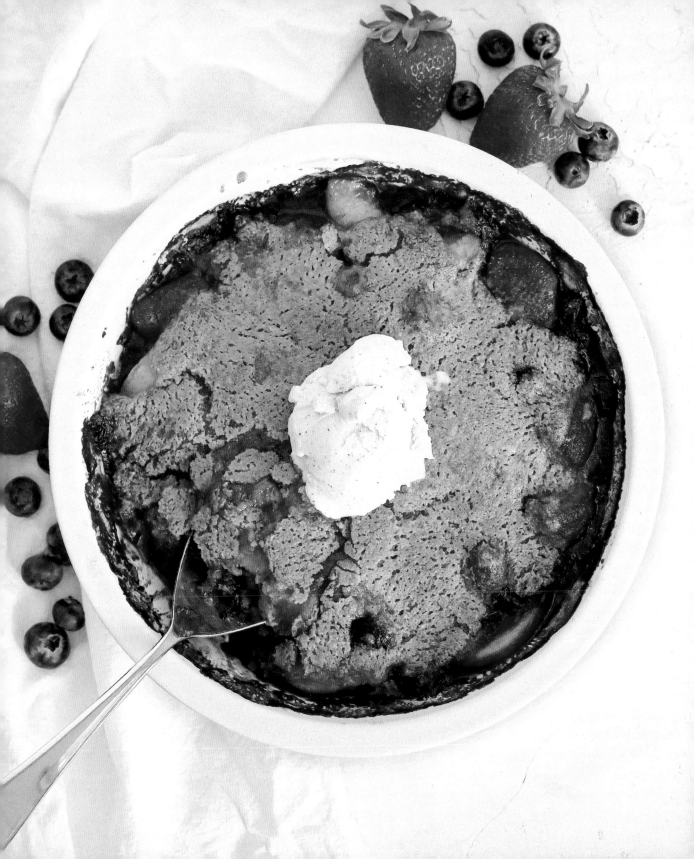

PEACH AND BERRY COBBLER

Cobbler is one of those desserts that looks fancy—almost as pretty as a pie—but is so simple to make. Use whatever fresh berries or stone fruits you have on hand, and bake them with the sweet, buttery cobbler topping until it's golden and bubbly. Serve this cobbler with dairy-free vanilla ice cream for the perfect crowd-pleasing dessert!

YIELD: 6 TO 8 SERVINGS

FILLING

Melted grass-fed butter or coconut oil, as needed

2 cups (300 g) fresh halved strawberries (see Note)

1½ cups (225 g) fresh blueberries

1 cup (225 g) thickly sliced fresh peaches

2 tbsp (16 g) arrowroot flour

2 tbsp (24 g) coconut sugar

TOPPING

¾ cup (72 g) almond flour

¼ cup (48 g) coconut sugar

¼ cup (60 g) grass-fed butter or coconut oil, melted

2 tbsp (30 ml) coconut milk

2 tbsp (16 g) arrowroot flour

1 tsp baking powder

1 tsp pure vanilla extract

¼ tsp salt

Dairy-free vanilla ice cream, as needed (optional)

1. To make the filling, preheat the oven to 375°F (191°C). Grease a 9-inch (23-cm) pie dish with the butter. Add the strawberries, blueberries and peaches to the dish. Add the arrowroot flour and sugar and toss the fruit to coat.

2. To make the topping, combine the almond flour, sugar, butter, coconut milk, arrowroot flour, baking powder, vanilla and salt in a small bowl and stir until the topping is smooth. Use a spoon to dollop the topping over the top of the berry mixture and smooth the top lightly.

3. Bake the cobbler for 25 to 30 minutes, or until the fruit is soft and the topping is light golden brown and set.

4. Serve the cobbler warm with dairy-free ice cream (if using).

NOTE: Fresh fruit works best for this recipe. If you are using frozen, thaw the fruit first and drain any excess moisture before adding it to the dish.

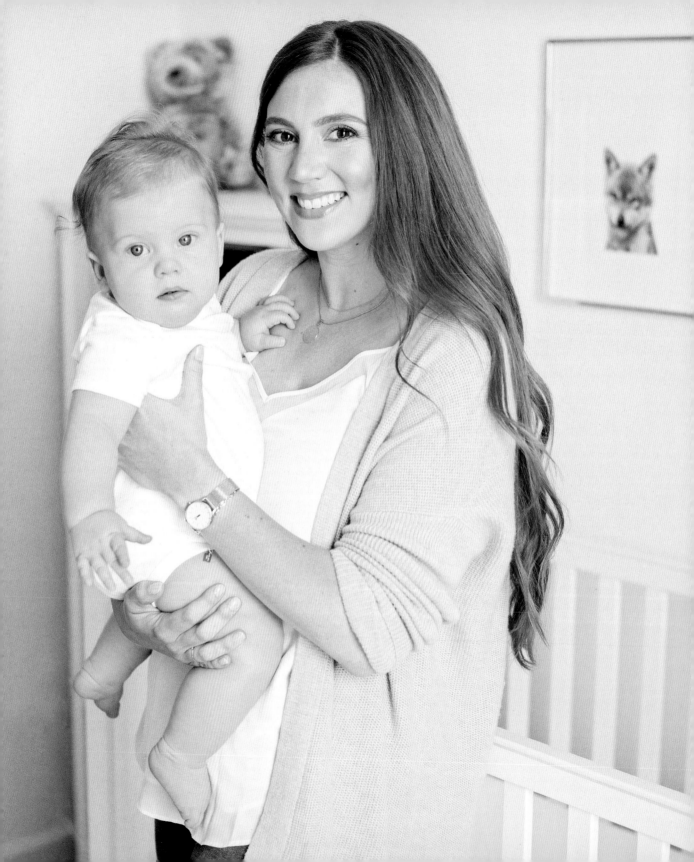

ACKNOWLEDGMENTS

To my boys, Hudson and Ford, for inspiring me to do big things and dream bigger than myself and what feels possible. You are my reason, my joy, my heart and my hope. Thank you for being here with me for this journey. I love you both so much, and I know you will do wonderful things if you set your minds to it.

To my husband, Dathan, for supporting my every dream without question and doing whatever it takes to make it happen. You are my rock, and none of this Just Jessie B stuff would have even begun if it weren't for your encouragement and unwavering belief in me and what I'm capable of. Thank you for supporting me year after year—and for being my best taste tester!

To my mom, for being my listening ear over every stress, my baby wrangler during recipe shoots and my best friend throughout every journey of this life. You have shown me just how it looks to "do it all," and I will forever aspire to be more like you.

To my dad, for teaching me to be resilient and always fight for what I want. You are my biggest example of how daily hard work and consistency truly pays off. Your endless love and support mean more to me than you know.

To my "little" brother, Alex, for eating all of the chicken tenders and pizza bites with me in our childhood. How boring my recipes would be today if I didn't have all of that for inspiration! Your moving into a grown-up home with a kitchen of your own has been one of my biggest inspirations for the simplicity of the recipes in this book.

To the team at Page Street Publishing, for believing in me and making my cookbook dream come true. It has been an honor to work with you all. Thank you for your guidance and expertise and for designing this beautiful book I am so proud of!

Finally, to my community of Just Jessie B readers and supporters: You all are the biggest reason this book has come to life, a dream I never thought I would see become reality. Thank you so much for trusting me, supporting me and welcoming me into your kitchens day after day. I love you all!

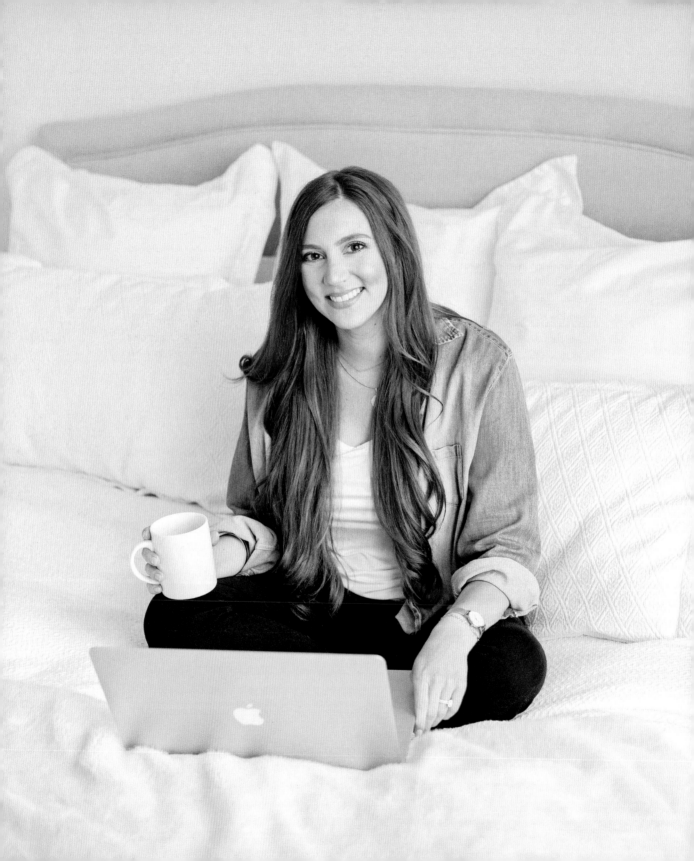

ABOUT THE AUTHOR

Jessie Bittner is the creator, blogger and photographer behind Just Jessie B, a food and lifestyle blog full of simple, mostly Paleo recipes and inspiration for living a clean and healthy life. She specializes in simple, comfort food–style, gluten- and dairy-free creations that the whole family will love—little ones and non-Paleo folks included.

Jessie's love for Paleo eating and cooking began in grad school, where she earned her master's degree in speech language pathology. She has spent several years following her other passion: working with children with special needs, including speech and language disorders.

Jessie now puts her love of food and helping children to work at home, running her own business and raising her two boys. Jessie lives in Morgan Hill, California, with her husband, Dathan, and their two boys, Hudson and Ford.

INDEX